Foundations in Nursing and Health Care

Profiles and Portfolios of Evidence

Ruth Pearce
Series Editor: Lynne Wigens

Published in 2003 by:
Nelson Thornes Ltd
Delta Place
27 Bath Road
CHELTENHAM
GL53 7TH
United Kingdom

05 06 07 / 10 9 8 7 6 5 4 3 2

A catalogue record for this book is available from the British Library

ISBN 0 7487 7123 9

Illustrations by Clinton Banbury
Page make-up by Florence Production Ltd.

Printed in Great Britain by Ashford Colour Press

Contents

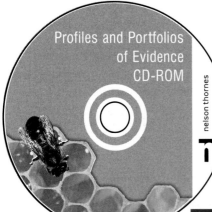

Profiles and Portfolios
of Evidence
CD-ROM

nelson thornes

What's on the CD-ROM

At the back of this book you will find a CD which provides you with templates and advice for creating your own portfolio. At various places in the book, you will find a CD icon in the margin such as appears here. This indicates a reference to information supplied on the CD or advice on how to use it. You will find instructions on how to run the CD on the disk body itself and once you open it, you will find a guidance file on how to use and adapt the material. The contents of the CD are listed below:

- CV guidelines
- CV template
- Job application letter
- Triangulation model
- Personal Development Plan
  - Personal Development Plan guidelines
  - Personal Development Plan template
  - Personal Development Plan example
- Continuing professional development model
- Reflective practice models
  - Gibbs's Reflective Cycle model and template
  - Johns's Reflective Model template
  - Palmer, Burns & Bulman's Reflective Model template
  - Goodman's Levels of Reflection
- Learning styles inventory
- Study day template
- Suggested portfolio structure.

However, if you prefer not to use the CD, there is more than enough information given in this book to help you create your own dynamic and professional portfolio.

1

Why do I need a professional portfolio?

Learning outcomes

By the end of this chapter you should be able to:

- Describe the historical development of professional portfolios
- Identify the purpose of a professional portfolio
- Identify the relevance of portfolio development for professional development
- Put the relevant work you have produced in your portfolio

Historical development

Health-care professional practice is difficult to define and can be difficult to learn; the subsequent training and assessment is equally problematic. Before the 1990s the majority of health-care professionals training focused on teaching routines and skills rather than on the ability to problem-solve, rationalise the care given and exercise individual professional judgement. There are many reasons as to why the education of health-care professionals has changed. The majority of these are driven by the government and the professional statutory bodies, who are responsible for implementing government policy. The increase in health-care technology and the culture of constant change that now seems synonymous with health care has influenced the need for increasingly competent and flexible professionals. With the increasing professionalisation of health-care practitioners it was deemed necessary for them to provide some evidence of responsibility for keeping themselves competent and up to date with their client care.

Hull and Redfern (1996) suggest that articles about the use of profiles and portfolios began to appear in British nursing and midwifery literature back in 1993. This suggestion is probably true of most health-care professions that now advocate the use of a professional portfolio. Nursing went a stage further in 1994 and the statutory body at the time, the United Kingdom Central Council (UKCC), now the Nursing and Midwifery Council (NMC), dictated that all nurses and midwives on the professional register needed to maintain a personal professional profile. From 1995, nurses and midwives wanting to re-register had to provide evidence in their personal professional profile that they had spent at least 5 days within the previous 3 years updating their knowledge and skills.

The Chartered Society of Physiotherapy (CSP) has produced a portfolio development guide that promotes continuing professional development and life-long learning, although it is not a requirement for registration as a physiotherapist. The Health Professions Council – which includes physiotherapists as well as dietitians, radiographers, etc. – is intending to introduce re-registration schemes in 2005, which could mean the submission of a portfolio for re-registration.

Portfolios have been around for a long time and portfolio development has been at the forefront of many professions such as art and architecture. In the arts a portfolio is used to display an artist's work in terms of depth, breadth, interest and abilities (Jongsma, 1989; Moya and O'Malley, 1994). Art and architect students have to prepare a portfolio and have always been inclined to carry their portfolios with them as an instant means of showing off their skills and talent in their field. Educators have used portfolios for a long time and there is now a move towards electronic portfolios. For example, traditionally, portfolios were assembled from collections of evidence stored in boxes or ring binders but they can now be stored in digital form. Students in the visual arts produce on-line portfolios, which are copied to CD-ROMs for distribution to other universities and potential employers.

Portfolio development in health care was introduced because of a change in health-care dynamics within the different professions. Health-care professions were forward-thinking and proactive in their introduction of portfolios. Arts, architecture and education had hitherto been the primary users of portfolios but the health-care professions were coming to realise the benefits of a portfolio as a medium for addressing the many variables within health care. For instance, nursing was changing from adherence to the biomedical model to a concept of health that incorporates economic, political, social, cultural, educational and ethical considerations. The support for the introduction of a portfolio was that it could address all the variables within health care, as it is very difficult to define client care and professional practice. The portfolio can bring together all the elements needed to demonstrate high-quality care and professional competence by providing evidence from multiple sources – practice, literature, study and research. Health-care professionals have to provide evidence of their competence and professional development to the clients, their statutory bodies and their employers. The portfolio was considered the most appropriate medium in which to express the diversity of practice and the professions.

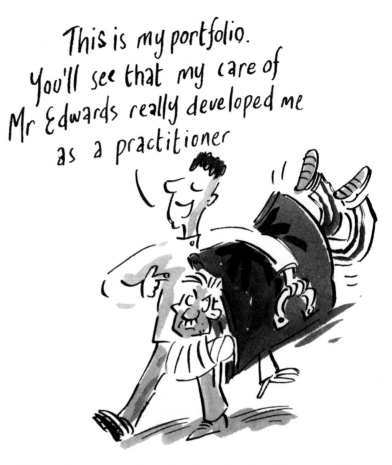

This is my portfolio. You'll see that my care of Mr Edwards really developed me as a practitioner

A portfolio provides a record of your development and growth as a practitioner

Key points | Top tips

A portfolio is used for different purposes:

- For health-care students a portfolio is often used in professional development and is assessed as part of their education and training.

- For qualified nurses the UKCC (now the Nursing and Midwifery Council) brought in legislation in 1995 that individuals on the professional register must use a personal professional profile. The profile is proof to the NMC that you, as an individual practitioner, are keeping yourself updated, maintaining competence and remaining accountable for your actions.

- The professional bodies of other health-care professionals, e.g. the Chartered Society of Physiotherapy, recommend the maintenance of a portfolio.

- The Health Professions Council (2003), the statutory regulatory body for allied health professionals, is intending to introduce re-registration schemes in 2005 that will relate to continuing professional development and how it is demonstrated, which could mean the submission of a portfolio for re-registration.

What is the purpose of a professional portfolio?

Perhaps before answering this question we need to ask what a portfolio is. Redman (1994) claims that it is simply a tangible record of what someone has done. It can also be described as a purposeful collection of materials that communicate your development. The words 'portfolio' and 'profile' seem to be interchangeable, and there has been some confusion as to whether they are the same thing or different. The NMC call the record a 'personal professional profile' and state that it is a record of career progress and professional development. The CSP call it a portfolio and use it to demonstrate continuing professional development and life-long learning. The Health Professions Council (2003) state that a **portfolio**:

- Is a resource (that can be a hard copy or electronic format) that helps professionals to record, evaluate and reflect on their learning
- Provides a tool for identifying ongoing learning needs and planning activity to meet these needs
- Can be used to support a range of purposes (including preparation for annual appraisals, applying for a new job and seeking academic credit for work based learning).

Hull and Redfern (1996) provide the definition of a **profile** as a selection of specific evidence for a specific purpose to present to a specific audience.

For the purposes of this book, what we are discussing will be called a portfolio, not a profile. Even when you present your portfolio for assessment or scrutiny at interview or to a professional body, I still believe that it is a portfolio, even although certain more personal accounts may have been removed.

Keywords

Portfolio
A collection of individual material that provides proof of personal growth, continuing professional development, life-long learning and competence

Keywords

Profile
A public version of the portfolio – a summary of your portfolio that can be offered at interview to support your application or can be submitted to professional bodies as proof of continuing professional development

Which is the best portfolio for you?

Which is the best portfolio for you really depends on how you feel about a portfolio and its purpose. You may feel that you are unsure how to collect and organise all the relevant information, so you may prefer to buy a ready-structured portfolio. There are many 'ready-made' portfolios on the market; it is not a requirement of any of the health-care professional bodies that you use a professionally produced portfolio, although the CSP do provide a CD-ROM to help you to develop your own. Alternatively, you may feel that you want the freedom to produce your own version, based on what you feel is relevant and how you learn best. Chapter 8 of this book provides examples of how you can structure your portfolio.

A basic version of a portfolio could take the form of a folder where you keep things related to your development, training, work experience and special activities. You may wonder why this is considered to be a basic portfolio when this is probably the definition you are currently working with. The description implies that the portfolio is a folder in which you keep important certificates or documents. It does not mention the real purpose of a portfolio, which is to reflect personal and professional growth and communicate your development through demonstrating self-awareness and reflection. It is undeniably a resource for all your work-related activity and educational development but it should, more importantly, provide you with an overall awareness of who and where you are as a practitioner. An effective portfolio is a visual representation of you and your experience, strengths, abilities and skills. The purpose of a portfolio from a professional and educational body viewpoint is to encourage:

- The development of self-assessment and self-reflective skills
- Documentation of continuing professional development, life-long learning and achievements
- Application of course content/theory to clinical experiences
- The attainment of learning outcomes
- Analysis, action planning and evaluation of learning needs.

Up until the late 1990s, practitioners universally used ring binders as their portfolios, whether 'ready-made' or self-assembled. In fact, many still do. This book provides you with a CD-ROM to help formulate your portfolio and you may question the benefits of a CD-ROM over a traditional folder portfolio. The general movement in portfolio development is towards electronic portfolios. E-portfolios, according to Barrett (2002), are essentially a new kind of 'container'. You will not be judged on the type of portfolio presentation you choose to use. Your choice will depend upon how comfortable you are with each type. If you are computer-literate, an e-portfolio may be more attractive to you than a folder one. Alternatively, you may like to see your work presented in a folder portfolio, as you may be more familiar with and prefer a paper version of such things.

When considering what type of portfolio presentation you prefer:

- Bear in mind what the portfolio is going to be used for
- For a student portfolio you may be given a portfolio and guidelines as to how it should be produced and presented
- For a portfolio for personal use, you have freedom to choose the type of presentation you prefer
- Remember that you might need the portfolio for interview and, if you have an e-portfolio, you cannot guarantee that the interviewer will have access to a computer – so ensure that you can print off any relevant sections necessary for the interview

How can a portfolio help me?

A portfolio can seem a bit overwhelming. In practical terms a portfolio is essential to demonstrate professional development, clinical competence and life-long learning. A portfolio can help by assisting you in self-awareness, through reflection and self-evaluation, and in empowerment, through analysis and critiquing your own work. It also provides you with evidence of:

- Reflections on academic and clinical experiences
- Continuing professional development and life-long learning
- Decisions about the quality of your work
- Effective critical thinking
- Reflection on professional growth
- Empowerment to take responsibility for your own learning
- Development towards being a critical, reflective practitioner
- Document achievements.

In addition:

- It can enhance self-esteem by focusing on accomplishments
- It can also help you to obtain a position/job promotion by demonstrating all of the above.

You need to start developing your portfolio from the day you start training. One of the aims of a student portfolio is to help you to progress from responsibility to accountability. You are **responsible** for your care and actions as a student but become **accountable** when you qualify.

A portfolio can seem quite an exciting prospect; it could read like an episode of a TV hospital drama, a vibrant mix of experience and relationships. Now consider your TV hospital drama episode in the

○━ᴚ *Keywords*

Responsible
Answerable for what you do

Accountable
Answerable for what you do **and** the consequences of what you do

context of academic assessment or professional requirements and it may seem less interesting.

Starting a portfolio can seem very daunting, especially if you feel you have either a great deal or very little experience of life so far. Whichever it is, you have already developed your own personal values and beliefs and a sense of what you feel is right or wrong. These personal beliefs and values are very important, especially when put alongside the professional values within which you work. One of the most difficult aspects of working in health care is the acknowledgement of your own personal beliefs and values and the recognition that they may be very different from the beliefs and values held by your clients and your peers.

Portfolio development for students is as important as for qualified practitioners. The student portfolio is the one medium where all aspects of a health-care course can be assessed as a whole. It represents all the clinical, theoretical and professional modules health-care courses offer and requires you to make links between the modules studied to **contextualise** the process of learning and continuing professional development.

Keywords

Contextualise
To put theory into an everyday, practical situation

RRRRR Rapid recap

Check your progress so far by working through each of the following questions.
1. What is a portfolio?
2. What is a profile?
3. What is the purpose of keeping a portfolio for:
    a) a health-care student
    b) a qualified practitioner?
If you have difficulty with any of the questions, read through the section again to refresh your understanding before moving on.

References

Barrett, H. (2002) *Directions in Electronic Portfolio Development*. Available online: www.electronicportfolios.com (accessed February 2003).

Health Professions Council (2003) Available online: www.healthprofessionscouncil.co.uk (accessed February 2003).

Hull, C. and Redfern, L. (1996) *Profiles and Portfolios: A guide for nurses and midwives*. Macmillan, Basingstoke.

Jongsma, K. S. (1989) Portfolio assessment. *Reading Teacher*, **43**, 264–265.

Moya, S. S. and O'Malley, J. M. (1994) A portfolio assessment model for ESL. *Journal of Educational Issues of Language Minority Students*, **13**, 13–36.

Redman, W. (1994) Portfolios for development. Kogan Page, London.

2

Linking theory to practice

Learning outcomes

By the end of this chapter you should be able to:

- Understand the development of a portfolio and the importance of linking theory, practice, education and research

- Recognise your preferred learning style and consider learning strategies to make the most of your learning experiences

- Contemplate how reflective learning from experience can enhance self-assessment and personal and pro-fessional development

As a health-care student you may find it difficult to define how you learn something. You may be aware how you learn best but are still unsure as to the subtleties of how you actually learn a skill. Learning a health-care profession presents itself in complicated and negotiated ways, which can lead to confusion and aspects of learning being fragmented. This can be reinforced by the disparate experiences in the clinical area compared to the university experience. The separation of theory and practice between the service providers and the university can often represent the differing, sometimes competitive forces driving both. Clinical areas, first and foremost, need competent practitioners who are safe and fit for practice; the universities provide competent practitioners but perhaps aspire to provide practitioners capable of being critical and rationalising the care given. While clinical areas obviously want practitioners capable of rationalising care, service providers are driven by a more pressing demand – to have safe and competent staff working in their Trusts as soon as possible.

Melia (1987) argues that a profession such as nursing is too diverse an enterprise and that the occupational group of nurses is too large and heterogeneous a group for its members to share the same view of what their work should be. This reflects the difficulty encountered by the NMC in ensuring standards. The main aim of a portfolio is a tentative attempt to unite the two and demonstrate how they inform each other.

Background to experiential learning theory

One of the biggest complaints I hear from students at university is that their education begins with a lot of theory. As a health-care student you have chosen a vocational course and want to begin practising as soon as possible. Many students struggle with a theoretical concept until it is applied in practice. If you find it difficult to learn in these circumstances it may be a result of the

○━┭ Keywords

Experiential learning
A type of learning that uses
reflection to inform practice
and learning, as every
individual learns differently
(Kolb, 1984)

teaching and learning approach rather than because you are unable to grasp the concept. If you find it difficult to learn when given theory first and practice later, you may prefer the **experiential learning** approach.

Universities recognise the need for experiential learning when providing a vocational course and many try to unite theory and practice by adopting a variety of teaching methods.

In this chapter you will identify your own experiential learning style and build on this information to help you better understand:

- How you make career choices
- How you solve problems
- How you set goals
- How you manage yourself and others
- How you deal with new situations.

Experiential learning can apply to any kind of learning through experience. The experiential learning model pursues a framework for examining and strengthening the critical linkages among education, work and personal development (Kolb, 1984). As you can see, these three main components that Kolb identifies link directly to the portfolio. The portfolio represents the merging of education, professional and personal development. Kolb (1984) suggests that the ability to learn is the most important skill we can acquire because we are often confronted with new experiences or learning situations in life, our careers, or on the job.

Principles of experiential learning

- Experiential learning recognises that people learn best from their own experiences and their own reviews
- Experiential learning subscribes to the notion that what people do is more important than what they know
- Experiential learning renders behaviours and attitudes visible and thereby can become acknowledged and then addressed
- Experiential learning is built on the premise that it is not enough to explain to people what to do, they must be shown how to actually do it and then how to improve it
- Experiential learning moves beyond knowledge and into skill by generating a learning experience – the more experience the greater the skill
- Experiential learning gets to grips with the most important aspect of training and that is to achieve change in behaviour and attitude
- Experiential learning understands that to be remembered over a long period of time the learning process should be enjoyable, motivating and rewarding

Experiential Learning (2003) www.teamskillstraining.co.uk

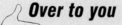

Over to you

Think about something new you've recently learnt. How did you learn it? Do you prefer to watch something being done or do you prefer to read about something first and then think about it? Note down the different stages involved in both these types of learning.

You probably find you have a preference as to how you learn best. Kolb (1984) considered these preferences and called them 'learning styles'. This may not seem particularly relevant – you may not have given it much thought before now – but knowing your learning style and how you learn best can focus your learning, identify your strengths and weaknesses and help in choosing what you might be good at.

There are different learning-style questionnaires that enable you to analyse your learning style; they are called learning style inventories. Kolb (1984) and Honey and Mumford (1986) seem to be the most popular learning-style inventories studied by health-care professionals. Within this book I will discuss Kolb's learning style inventory but it is equally valid for you to do the Honey and Mumford learning style inventory as well as or instead of Kolb – the CSP, for example, recommends Honey and Mumford.

Kolb recognised two learning actions: perception and processing. He then divided the actions into opposites. So in the area of perception, if you learn best by watching something you prefer learning from *concrete experience*. If you prefer to think theoretically, you prefer what is termed *conceptualisation*.

Once you have received the information, you then have to deal with it, which is the processing element of the learning action. If you enjoy learning from concrete experiences you may prefer to use the information in a practical way, *active experimentation*, while others perceive best by thinking about the information they have received, *reflective observation*.

In order to be an effective learner it is useful to be able to adopt all the learning actions mentioned but you will find there will be a type of learning you favour, and learn best from.

There are four dimensions in Kolb's learning cycle (Figure 2.1):

● Concrete experience
  – Getting involved and learning from specific experiences related to people
● Reflective observation
  – Describing the experience itself
  – Critically analysing the experience

- Creating a new conception and knowledge
- Listening and observing before making a judgement; you view things from different perspectives and look for the meaning of things

● Abstract conceptualisation
- Creating and analysing ideas; systematic planning

● Active experimentation
- Getting things done and making decisions
- Displaying leadership skills and influencing people
- Occasionally involves taking risks.

Look at the cycle again and try to decide where you fit. If you fit between Active Experimentation and Concrete Experience you are predominantly an *Accommodator.* If you fit between concrete experience and reflective observation you are a *Diverger.* If you fall between reflective observation and abstract conceptualisation you are an *Assimilator* and finally if you fall between abstract conceptualisation and active experimentation you are a *Converger.* An individual with an abstract learning style such as a Converger can learn to communicate ideas more effectively by associating with individuals who are more concrete and people-oriented, such as the Diverger. Individuals with a more reflective learning style (Diverger/Assimilator) can link with someone who is more active in their style of learning like the Accommodator.

Accommodator

You are primarily a 'hands-on' learner – you like to carry out plans. You prefer other people's analysis to your own and act on intuition. You enjoy a challenge and applying your learning in real life situations.

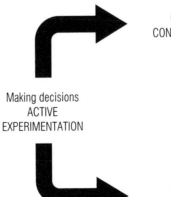
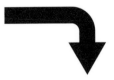
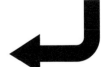

Getting involved
CONCRETE EXPERIENCE

Listening
REFLECTIVE
OBSERVATION

Making decisions
ACTIVE
EXPERIMENTATION

Creating an idea
ABSTRACT CONEPTUALISATION

Figure 2.1 *Kolb's learning cycle*

Diverger

You like to look at things from different points of view. You prefer to watch rather than take action. You like to gather information and are good at coming up with ideas. You like using your imagination in problem-solving and are quite sensitive.

Assimilator

You tend to solve problems and are rational. You are less bothered by social interaction and prefer technical tasks.

Converger

You are concise and logical and good at finding solutions. Problem solving is more important to you than people issues. Practicality is less important to you than a good logical explanation.

Identifying your learning style

This questionnaire is designed to find out your preferred learning style(s). It was first designed by David Kolb in 1970. There is no time limit to this questionnaire but it will probably take about 10–15 minutes. There are no right or wrong answers. Look at the four statements in each row, and decide how they refer to you. Give four marks to the statement nearest to you, three to the second, two for the third and one for the statement least like you.

Use the grid in Table 2.2 to summarise your score on the Learning Style inventory and fill in your total score for each column in the spaces below.

Now use the scores you have from the four columns in the following way.

First, subtract your RO score from your AE score.

Second, subtract your CE score from your AC score.

Plot the resulting figures on the two axes in Figure 2.2.

The four scores you originally arrived at can be plotted on to Figure 2.3 and joined up to produce your 'kite'.

The shape of your kite gives you a profile of your learning style and the ways in which you are likely to learn best.

There are many ways in which we can plan to work with our learning style once we have analysed it. It helps us to know how we learn best and how others learn. It is good practice to try to learn from a variety of teaching and learning methods but most practitioners will find they learn best using one or two particular methods. As part of your development you can aim to work on learning from different methods from the one you favour. This will

Table 2.1 The learning style inventory (Kolb, 1984)

	a	b	c	d
1	I like to get involved	I like to take my time before acting	I am particular about what I like	I like things to be useful
2	I like to try things out	I like to analyse things and break them down into parts	I am open to new experiences	I like to look at all sides of issues
3	I like to watch	I like to follow my feelings	I like to be doing things	I like to think about things
4	I accept people and situations the way they are	I like to be aware of what is around me	I like to evaluate	I like to take risks
5	I have gut feelings and hunches	I have a lot of questions	I am logical	I am hard working and get things done
6	I like concrete things I can see, feel, touch and smell	I like to be active	I like to observe	I like ideas and theories
7	I prefer learning in the here and now	I like to consider and reflect about them	I tend to think about the future	I like to see the results of my work
8	I have to try things out for myself	I rely on my own ideas	I rely on my own observations	I rely on my own feelings
9	I am quiet and reserved	I am energetic and enthusiastic	I tend to reason things out	I am responsible about things

Table 2.2 Scoring grid for learning styles inventory

CE Concrete experience	RO Reflective observation	AC Abstract conceptualisation	AE Active experimentation
1a	1b	2b	2a
2c	2d	3d	3c
3b	3a	4c	6b
4a	6c	6d	7d
8d	8c	8b	8a
9b	9a	9c	9d
Total	**Total**	**Total**	**Total**

Only put down the 'marks' asked for. You will notice that the marks for 1c and 1d are not asked. This is intended to stop 'patterning' and is not a mistake.

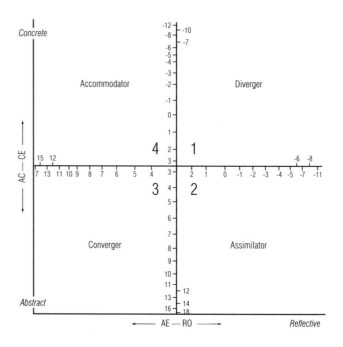

Figure 2.2 *Axis diagram*

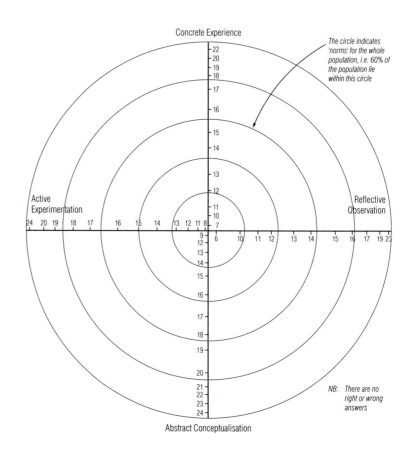

Figure 2.3 *Kite diagram*

demonstrate increased perception of how you learn and the need to enhance your repertoire of learning and skill development.

Understanding your learning style helps in developing awareness of strengths in some steps of the learning cycle and can assist you in:

- Choosing a career path
- Problem solving
- Managing people
- Working as part of a team (Kolb and Joyce, 1995).

Within the Learning Styles Inventory is a career map, in which Kolb and Joyce (1995) highlight areas to which each learning style is most suited. A Diverger is considered the most relevant learning type for many of the health-care professions but you need to remember that within each health-care profession there are many specialities. Each of these professions needs a manager, teacher, administrator and researcher.

How is knowing your learning style going to help you?

Knowing how you learn best can provide you with the strategies you need to develop your learning and enhance your problem solving skills. As mentioned already, each health-care profession will have representatives from each learning style. This is important in building an effective team and learning how to work together. Kolb and Joyce (1995) recommend that you develop relationships with people whose learning style is different from your own. The point of this is to provide you with an insight into how other people learn and what strategies they use. For example, as an Accommodator you may struggle with reflective practice and consequently with portfolio development, as you find it more difficult to analyse how you learn. Working with a Diverger or Assimilator could help you to appreciate the need to reflect and the process of learning from reflection. Now you can opt to modify how you learn by adapting learning that is presented to you so that it more closely matches your preferred style and become even more proficient in your preferred style. If you can develop this awareness, you can take it one step further by becoming what Kolb and Joyce (1995) term a 'flexible learner'. This involves working on the weaknesses in your learning style so you can develop your learning and problem-solving skills. This can be very difficult, especially if you don't enjoy learning a particular way, but it does provide you with a greater appreciation of learning and how others learn and will help you become a flexible learner.

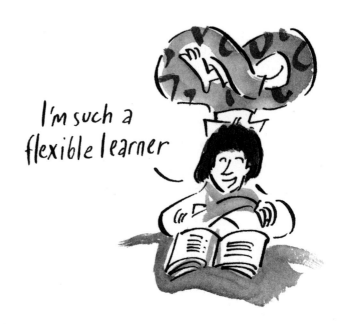

Being flexible in your learning will aid your development

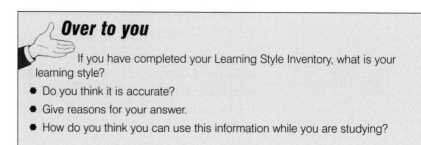

Over to you

If you have completed your Learning Style Inventory, what is your learning style?

● Do you think it is accurate?

● Give reasons for your answer.

● How do you think you can use this information while you are studying?

Now that you know your learning style you can develop strategies to aid your learning.

Kolb's experiential learning cycle can also be used to describe or reflect on an experience.

Using Kolb's experiential learning cycle helped Kerry (in the Case study on the next page) to reflect on an experience and come up with strategies to deal with the situation if it arose again. She also created a worthwhile idea for her mentor to consider to improve her practice and emphasise the message she was trying to communicate.

Not all authors believe that experiential learning cycles are enough in terms of supporting and charting student learning and progress. Nicklin and Kenworthy (2000) warn that the term 'experiential learning' can sometimes be misinterpreted

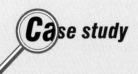

Case study

Kerry's experiential learning

Kerry is a student dietician using Kolb's learning cycle to demonstrate her experiential learning.

Concrete experience

I was gathering information regarding the eating habits of children and my mentor had been invited to talk to a mother and toddler group about nutrition in children.

Reflective observation

The talk was given in the morning and there were snacks (biscuits) and drinks out on tables for the children. During the talk my mentor suggested that instead of a plate of biscuits as a mid-morning snack they put a plate of fruit out or packets of raisins to encourage the children to eat fruit. One of the mothers was trying to feed her child an apple but because the child could see a plate of biscuits he refused to eat the apple. I witnessed the mother smack her child as he spat a piece of the apple out that she had forced into his mouth. She then made him sit down next to a plate of biscuits and look at them but not touch them. I felt really sorry for the little boy, he only wanted what all the other children in the room had. Denying the child a snack only made him bad-tempered and lethargic. Sitting the child down in front of the biscuits only created stress for her and for the little boy and I don't think the little boy learned anything from the experience. Professionally, I think she was trying to uphold the principles of a good diet and normally I would applaud such a mother but I felt her desire to prove she gave her child fruit and not biscuits was inappropriate and cruel.

Creating ideas

I felt if the mother objected so strongly to the biscuits she should have taken the child away so as not to leave temptation in his path. Rather than sitting him in front of the biscuits she could have distracted him by letting him play with the other toddlers and just said a quiet and firm 'No' if he went to take a biscuit. I suggested to my mentor that the next time we went to give a talk to a playgroup we suggested the organiser of the playgroup provide a plate of fruit to enhance the message we were trying to get across. It seemed a bit ironic to be talking about and providing literature on eating fresh fruit and vegetables when the children were eating biscuits and highly coloured juice.

Active experimentation

I didn't get to attend another talk to a playgroup but my mentor did say she would take on board my idea and ask the organiser of the next playgroup to provide fresh fruit if possible.

Keywords

Experiential taxonomy
A rational framework suited to competence-based education and training

as purely 'self-awareness' training. They consider that an **experiential taxonomy** is better structured than experiential learning, as they believe that experiential learning can be simply a learning strategy.

The experiential taxonomy they use was devised and developed by Steinaker and Bell (1979) and comprises five levels:

- **Exposure level**: The student is introduced to and is conscious of an experience
- **Participation level**: The student has to make a decision to become part of the experience
- **Identification level**: The student identifies with the experience both intellectually and emotionally
- **Internalisation level**: The student progresses to this level when the experience begins to affect daily life, changing behaviours and ways of doing things
- **Dissemination level**: The student now expresses the experience, advocating it to others.

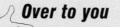

Over to you

Think about a recent experience you have had and relate it to Steinaker and Bell's experiential taxonomy.
Try to identify the different levels and which level you felt you were at.
Then try and identify what further experience or knowledge would help you to progress to the dissemination level.

What the taxonomy promotes is what educationalists term 'deep' learning. With any kind of learning, the approach to learning is very important. Ramsden (1992) discusses various approaches to learning especially the 'how' and the 'what' of learning.

The 'how' of learning is the construct, as in the act of experiencing, organising and structuring, and this can be done two ways – using the holistic approach, which focuses on the whole in relation to the parts, and using the atomistic approach, which focuses on the parts as segments of the whole.

The 'what' of learning is looking for the meaning of what is experienced and can be subdivided into two approaches: deep and surface learning. Deep learning focuses on what the experience is about and surface learning focuses on the basic elements of the experience without any linking beyond the experience itself.

The ultimate aim of any educational process, whether it is portfolio development or an assignment or care study, is for the student or practitioner to demonstrate meaningful learning through using a holistic and deep approach. For example, you have probably used surface learning for studying during exams by cramming the night before to gather and then recall as much information as possible during the exam. With this approach you probably find that after the exam you have little recollection of the information you spent the night before cramming. Deep learning is when you integrate all the information you have received, either through teaching sessions, observing practice, participating in practice, reading or discussions. You develop a deeper understanding of the key issues and can then use this knowledge at a later date and apply it to different situations, thus enabling problem solving.

Entwistle (1997) states that the intention of a deep approach to learning is to understand ideas for yourself by relating ideas to previous knowledge and experience, looking for underlying principles, checking evidence and relating it to conclusions, and examining logic and argument cautiously and critically. In comparison, the surface approach to learning is described as the intention to cope with requirements such as those arising from an academic course or a professional body. This involves studying without reflecting on either purpose or strategy and treating course or professional requirements as bits of knowledge. Ultimately Entwistle (1997) claims that the surface approach to learning will mean that you will find difficulty in making sense of new ideas and may feel undue pressure and worry about work.

You will be able to recall the feelings of stress and worry that you experienced when put in a situation you felt unprepared for. This can be similar to the experience of surface learning, as you have not prepared yourself adequately for the task in hand.

Obviously, even with a deep approach to learning you cannot prepare yourself for all the eventualities of practice. However, if you have fostered a deep approach to your learning you will have developed an understanding of the principles and can relate these to other experiences. You also have the skills to adapt and respond to whatever the experience demands.

By considering the deep and surface approaches to learning you should now have a greater appreciation of the purpose and potential of a portfolio. The portfolio should be considered as a whole, as it should demonstrate learning from a variety of contexts to provide an overview of you and who you are personally and professionally. A portfolio created using a surface approach will appear disjointed, as there will be little evidence of transferring and transforming knowledge, linking theory to practice and developing as a professional and competent practitioner. A portfolio is the one medium where you draw on an assortment of learning experiences to provide evidence of increasing knowledge, professional growth, enhanced skills and competence and application of knowledge to practice.

Reflective practice

Reflection is an effective tool for recognising formal and informal learning and development through practice and is particularly useful in the development of a portfolio. Kolb (1984) relates the process of reflection to experiential learning theory, which emphasises the value of critically evaluating experience as a learning action. Kolb identifies three stages of learning entrenched in reflection:

- The experience itself, which provides a base for reflection on observation

- Critical analysis of the experience, which develops and generates insight

- A new conception and knowledge of the experience which can be tested in new situations.

The term 'reflection' is not clearly defined. Boud *et al.* (1985) state that reflection is a generic term coined to describe those intellectual and affective activities in which individuals engage to explore their experiences in order to lead to new understanding and appreciation. These intellectual and affective activities are applied by individuals when they look back at an experience and reconstruct, re-enact and recapture the event, the emotions, the feelings, the thoughts and the accomplishment.

Three factors are intrinsic to the concept of reflection (Boyd and Fales, 1983):

- Action

- Critical thought

- The self.

Boyd and Fales (1983) state that reflective learning emphasises the self as the source of learning, the process of creating and clarifying the meaning of experience (present or past) in terms of self (self in relation to self and self in relation to the world). The outcome of the process is a changed conceptual perspective. The meaning focuses on or embodies a concern of central importance to the self. Donald Schon (1987) distinguishes between two types of reflection:

- **Reflection-in-action** is a dynamic process, the intuitive art of 'thinking on your feet', which occurs while practising and influences the decisions made and care given

- **Reflection-on-action** is a retrospective process, which occurs after the event and contributes to the development of practical skills.

The essential qualities of a portfolio include reflective practice, personal development plans, life-long learning and professional competence. A portfolio provides a medium for recording learning from practice and practice from learning. Gibbs (1988) believes that it is not enough just to have an experience in order to learn. Without reflecting on the experience it may be quickly forgotten and its learning potential will be lost. Conversely, practice cannot be changed just from learning; new concepts need to be tried out to link theory with practice. Reflection is of great importance in the professional life of a health-care professional and we all do it automatically, but perhaps not systematically, in our heads – the challenge for most health-care professionals is to write it down and learn from it.

Flexibility is the key to health-care practice. Health-care practice is known for its unpredictability and therefore you need to know how you handle diverse situations. You need to start developing strategies that will enable you to function effectively in such situations. This is why fostering a deep approach to your learning will enable you to develop these strategies, as you will be able to relate to previous knowledge and experience. As you develop as a competent practitioner you will have support from many different people, but you can help yourself through knowing how to recognise and deal with your own reactions. By reflecting on your clinical experiences you will know how you have dealt with challenges previously. You can then make action plans to predict and prevent the situation happening again.

Over to you

You need to determine the reflective model that suits you and your way of thinking. Examples of reflective models are given on the next few pages. Try each one and find which one you feel works through your experience and draws the most out of it. Structured reflective models do have their limitations and you will discover this as you use them. You may find that the cue questions just don't ask you for the key point or that you are completing the questions as a task rather than using a truly reflective approach. If you find they don't cover everything you wanted to say, add anything extra you want to but try to stay within the broad framework of the model, as Johns (1996) believes reflection needs to be guided. Conversely if you feel they ask too many questions, you can omit some of the questions but this would benefit by being supported by reasoning as to why you don't think the question is applicable.

Gibbs's reflective cycle

Gibbs's reflective cycle enables participants to practise the skills of reflection:

- Self-awareness
- Feelings
- Attitudes.

Stages of:

- Association
- Integration
- Validation
- Appropriation.

The need for:

- Description
- Analysis
- Synthesis
- Evaluation.

Gibbs's model is useful for less experienced staff or students as it directs you and offers an easy framework to use. Introducing a model of this type can support the introduction of reflection and the

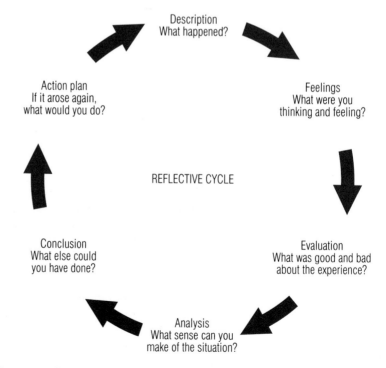

Figure 2.4 *Gibbs's reflective cycle (Gibbs, 1988)*

transition from student to practitioner. With experience, you may find this model a bit restrictive, but it is an excellent starting point for reflection.

Johns's holistic model

Johns's (1998) holistic model uses one core question such as aesthetics or ethics and then provides several reflective cue questions in order to direct practitioners to explore their experiences. The model is considered holistic as it looks beyond the traditional 'medical model' and encompasses wider aspects of social, cultural and psychological caring.

Aesthetics

- What was I trying to achieve?
- Why did I respond as I did?
- What was the consequence for patients and others?
- What were their feelings?
- How did I know this?

Personal

- How did I feel in this situation?
- What internal factors were influencing me?

Ethics

- How did my actions match my beliefs?
- What factors made me act in incongruent ways?

Empirics

- What knowledge informed me?

Reflexivity

- How does this connect with previous experiences?
- Could I handle this better in similar situations?
- What would be the consequence of alternative actions?
- How do I now feel about this experience?
- Can I support myself and others better as a consequence?
- Has this changed my ways of knowing?

•━┓ Keywords

Aesthetics
How you grasp and interpret the situation

•━┓ Keywords

Ethics
Doing the right thing – moral principles

Empirics
Using experience and knowledge to inform practice

Reflexivity
Acknowledges that an experience is not an isolated moment

> ## Over to you
>
> Using firstly Gibbs's and then Johns's reflective model reflect on a recent learning experience, link it to what you already knew or understood about your learning.
> - Which model did you prefer?
> - Can you put into words why you preferred one model over the other?

| **Top tips**

- Be careful when reflecting not to use the reflection as a means of off-loading all your frustrations regarding an experience. You need to stay objective and rational throughout. A good piece of advice is to focus on you and how you felt about the experience. A reflective piece that predominantly focuses on the feelings and actions of the other participants does not provide enough insight into you and how you dealt with a particular situation. Reflecting on practice is a process of self-reflection and should demonstrate this. Read Sanjay's reflection in the following Case study.

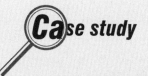

Case study

Sanjay's second-year reflection

Sanjay uses Gibbs's reflective cycle to reflect on his clinical placement during his second year.

Description: What happened?

An elderly lady had been having physiotherapy and had missed her lunch. She was quite frail and was on a food chart as she had problems relating to poor nutrition. She arrived back on the ward and didn't say anything about missing lunch as she had a poor appetite. I was on a late shift and went round checking the charts and chatting to the patients while the qualified members of staff were in 'report'. I noticed the patient had nothing filled in under lunch. I checked with my colleagues to see if she'd had lunch in case she had but it had not been recorded. My colleagues said she had not had any lunch. No lunch had been saved for her. I later discovered that one of the staff nurses had eaten a patient lunch thinking they were spare; this is against Trust policy. I contacted the kitchens but they said she could only have a sandwich as all hot meals had been cleared away. This was the only hot meal the patients are offered during the day.

Feelings: What were you thinking and feeling?

I felt a bit angry that no-one had thought to save the patient a lunch, especially as she was on a food chart and nutrition was one of her main problems. I also felt angry that a staff nurse had eaten a lunch when the patient needed one and this was against Trust policy. I felt annoyed that such a large Trust cannot provide a hot meal for a patient after a certain time and this meant the patient would not receive another hot meal that day. The kitchens can provide staff with a hot meal, so why not the patients? The whole episode also took me over an hour to resolve which meant I was late doing the observations, which made the staff nurse cross, I felt this was unfair as I was trying to look after the patient.

Evaluation: What was good and bad about the experience?

The experience was good as I did quite a bit of 'detective' work, working through the problem. The patient wasn't especially hungry and would not have admitted she had missed lunch as she didn't want to cause a fuss. She appreciated the trouble I went to to get her something she'd like to eat. I felt I'd accomplished something when she ate her sandwich and yoghurt.

The experience was bad because I felt angry that my colleagues had

Case study continued

Analysis: What sense can you make of this situation?

This I find quite difficult to do as there are several factors involved. The government claim they want a patient-centred NHS yet one of the most basic human needs is not being met due to cost cutting. According to the more senior staff on the ward, patients used to get offered hot meals three times a day but when the hospitals became Trusts and catering was put out to 'tender' the cheapest way of providing food is to have one hot meal at lunchtime and then the cold meals can be prepared in advance, therefore, reducing staffing levels during unsociable hours and also the cost of providing and heating hot food. I realise you can argue as to how many hot meals would this lady have at home ordinarily, but she had a debilitating illness, leaving her weak and undernourished.

My colleagues had been busy that day and missing the patient's lunch was really just an oversight but I felt it was crucial although it wasn't an everyday occurrence. The lateness of the physiotherapy appointment didn't help and this may need to be looked at..

Conclusion: What else could you have done?

I don't think there was much else I could have done. I think if I'd explained more fully to the staff nurse why I hadn't managed to do the other patients' observations she might have been less cross and more understanding, but sometimes when I get a bee in my bonnet about something I don't think to explain what I'm doing to the others affected by my actions.

Action Plan: If it arose, what would you do?

If the situation arose again I would do my best to alter the physiotherapy appointments. I realise this would be very difficult as it may just have been a one off, a physio may have been sick or they may have had extra patients, it was probably something that couldn't be avoided. I would suggest to the nurse in charge (if I felt brave enough!) that staff needed reminding about not eating patient food. I would also check out the Trust website to see if there was anywhere for staff or user comments on the Trust and I would bring up my concerns regarding the availability of hot meals outside 'regular' hours.

This is a good reflection, especially as Sanjay has started to look beyond day-to-day practice and has considered the current NHS structures and health economics in relation to the provision of food. This reflection is of a good standard for a second-year student and adequately represents Goodman's level 2 (see below). To improve the reflection or to raise it to Goodman's level 3, Sanjay could have brought in current literature to support his reflection. In other words, he could have found an article discussing the importance of nutrition for hospitalised patients or issues around the provision of health care. This would have added weight to his reflection and would have demonstrated his depth of knowledge, attained by having read around the subject.

Goodman's levels of reflections

As a guide to reflection, Goodman (1984) described differing levels of reflection, which describe the content of the reflection and the concerns it addresses. Goodman's levels of reflection can be applied within a reflective model. This may sound confusing but try and think about it a bit like Lego. Imagine that you are 3 years old and you are asked to build a tower with Lego. You can only build a basic tower because your knowledge of what towers are like is limited. You grow up a bit and are asked to build another tower. This time you can build a better tower, with a bit more attention to detail – perhaps a door and a window – as you have more knowledge of what a tower should look like. Then you're an adult and by this time the tower is probably quite complex, with a battlement or two. In this analogy the Lego tower corresponds to the levels of reflection: both are influenced by age/knowledge of the world or, in the case of the portfolio, experience. As a first-year student you would not be expected to produce a reflection that included detailed insights into professional goals and broader social structures, as you do not have the experience to provide you with these. However, if you are an experienced practitioner, a reflection should include these insights and others beyond them.

For your portfolio, once you have found a reflective model you are comfortable with, then apply the levels of reflection:

- **First level**: Reflection to reach given objectives – criteria for reflection are limited to technocratic issues of efficiency, effectiveness and accountability

- **Second level**: Reflection on the relationship between principles and practice – there is an assessment of the implications and consequences of actions and beliefs as well as the underlying rationale for practice.

- **Third level**: Reflection which besides the above incorporates ethical and political concerns – issues of justice and emancipation enter deliberations over the value of professional goals and practice and the practitioner makes links between the setting of everyday practice and broader social structure and forces.

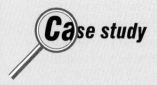

Case study

Jean's dilemma

Jean was a student physiotherapist and witnessed Mark, a qualified chest physiotherapist, about to treat a client without wearing an apron. Jean was unsure as to whether Mark had just forgotten or whether he didn't need to wear an apron. Recently she had had a lecture on cross-infection and was worried about the risks for the client and other clients Mark would be treating. She opted to make a definite point of putting an apron on but Mark did not notice, so she then asked him why he didn't wear an apron. It turned out that he had simply forgotten and thanked Jean for reminding him.

> ## Over to you
>
> Using a reflective model of your choice and pretending to be Jean, consider how you could write up this case study as a reflective piece.
> Give consideration to the different levels of reflection identified by Goodman (1984) in the light of Jean's case study.

By using a reflective approach to your learning you will generate your own values and beliefs, which are very important to your professional practice. It is these values and beliefs that make you the practitioner you are and this is what needs to be communicated through your portfolio. Recognition of others' values and beliefs is also very important, especially the values and beliefs of your clients. As health-care practitioners you will work with a mentor or clinical supervisor at some point in your career. These practitioners often act as very good role models and they are the people who often help shape the way you develop and create your values and beliefs.

Health-care professionals and students learn in many different ways and all learning is linked to clinical experience. The types of learning listed in the box below embody professional practice and provide the learner with evidence of how personal and professional development can be demonstrated.

⊶ Keywords

Triangulation of evidence
Drawing on three aspects of professional practice (experience, theory and evidence) in order to support the evidence in your portfolio

Learning for practice	Professional development courses/modules
	Study/theory days
Learning while practicing	Personal and professional development through reflection
	Personal development plans
	Teaching/mentoring/shadowing
	Reflection-in-action
	Reflection-on-action
Learning through practice	Evidence-based practice
	Practice based projects/research
	Learning sets

All the aspects of learning for practice, while practising and through practice can be demonstrated within the portfolio and this is really what it should include. If you can demonstrate all the above you are providing the **triangulation of evidence**, discussed in Chapter 3, as a reliable standard of what evidence in your portfolio should include.

One of the major problems you might experience with portfolio development is the lack of time you have to complete reflective entries and think about your experiences in depth. The concept of reflection is embedded within professional practice and most healthcare curricula, although this is not always the perception of healthcare professionals and students. A portfolio is often considered to be an additional and unnecessary piece of work, rather than an essential part of professional practice. The value of reflection, despite it being seen as an essential requirement of today's practitioner, is often undervalued.

ℛℛℛℛℛ*Rapid recap*

Check your progress so far by working through each of the following questions.
1. What are the four dimensions in Kolb's Learning Cycle?
2. What is 'deep learning'?
3. According to Schon, what is the difference between reflection-in-action and reflection-on-action?

If you have difficulty with any of the questions, read through the section again to refresh your understanding before moving on.

References

Boud, D., Keogh, R. and Walker, D. (1985) *Reflection: Turning experience into learning*. Kogan Page, London.

Boyd, E.M. and Fales, A.W. (1983) Reflective learning: key to learning from experience. *Journal of Humanistic Psychology*, **23**, 99–117.

Entwistle, N.J. (1997) *The Experience of Learning: Implications for teaching and studying in higher education*, 2nd edn. Scottish Academic Press, Edinburgh.

Experiential Learning (online) 2003 Available from www.teamskillstraining.co.uk/tst_article1.htm#teambuilding2 (accessed 6 February 2003).

Gibbs, G. (1988) *Learning by Doing: A guide to teaching and learning methods*. Further Education Unit, Oxford Polytechnic, Oxford.

Goodman, J. (1984) Reflection and teacher education: a case study and theoretical analysis. *Interchanges*, **15**, 9–26.

Honey, P. and Mumford, A. (1986) *Manual of Learning Styles*. P. Honey, Maidenhead, Berkshire.

Johns, C. (1996) Visualizing and realizing caring in practice through guided reflection. *Journal of Advanced Nursing* **24**, 1135–1143.

Johns, C. (1998) Opening the doors of perception, in *Transforming Nursing Through Reflective Practice* (eds C. Johns and D. Freshwater). Blackwell Science, Oxford.

Kolb, D. (1984) *Experiential Learning as the Science of Learning and Development*. Prentice Hall, Englewood Cliffs, NJ.

Kolb, D.A. and Joyce, S. (1995) Organisational behaviour: an experiential approach, 6th edn. Prentice Hall, London.

Melia, K. (1987) *Learning and Working: The occupational socialisation of nurses.* Tavistock Publications, London.

Nicklin, P. and Kenworthy, N. (2000) *Teaching and Assessing in Nursing Practice*, 3rd edn. Baillière Tindall, London.

Ramsden, P (1992) *Learning to Teach in Higher Education*. Routledge, London.

Schon, D.A. (1987) *Educating the Reflective Practitioner*. Jossey-Bass, San Francisco, CA.

Steinaker, N. and Bell, R. (1979) *The Experiential Taxonomy: A new approach to teaching and learning*. Academic Press, New York.

How to plan and produce your portfolio

Learning outcomes

By the end of this chapter you should be able to:

- Consider what evidence is needed to begin your portfolio
- Demonstrate understanding of how to inform your portfolio development in relation to your learning style
- Identify the relevance of produced evidence to individual learning needs
- Identify the relevance of produced evidence in relation to client care and best practice.

•⚷ *Keywords*

....

Prescriptive
Laying down rules

Beginning

Getting started is the most difficult aspect of portfolio development. Often, portfolio development is very different from other forms of learning you have experienced and the difference in the learning can be the first stumbling block. Portfolio guidelines are usually not **prescriptive** and have a degree of flexibility, which can add to the confusion of how to develop one. This chapter will help to provide more concrete guidelines and make the purpose of a portfolio and the subsequent learning more enjoyable.

Envisage the portfolio as a frame without a picture; the picture most academic institutions and professional bodies want to see is a self-portrait. You need to provide the self-portrait to fill the frame. It is the portrait that provides the depth, warmth and interest, not the frame. It is you who provide the essence. The portfolio should be about you and your professional life, the things you like to do and do best, what makes you the practitioner you are, what experiences have shaped your way of thinking. Chapter 1 discussed the fact that the portfolios produced by artists and architects are intended to exhibit the depth, breadth, interest and abilities they possess. This is applicable to your own portfolio – ensure that it is a true representation of you and your abilities.

Structuring a portfolio

The content of a portfolio depends on its purpose. If the portfolio is for assessment purposes, you will be given clear guidelines on what it should contain, or at least be given learning outcomes that can guide your content. With a generic portfolio, there is much more freedom in terms of what you can include. Next is a list of personal and professional activities that are appropriate in the context of a portfolio and can represent a portfolio inventory.

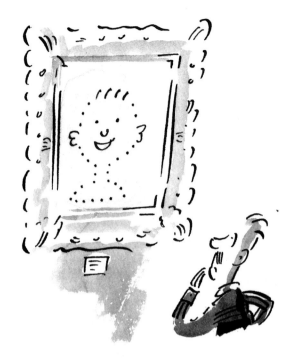

Your portfolio should represent who and what you are

Portfolio inventory

Work-related activities
- Curriculum vitae
- Performance reports, appraisals (e.g. personal tutor meetings, mentor appraisals, continuous assessment of practice documents)
- Letter of nomination and/or recommendation
- Accomplishments (could include newspaper clippings that detail your achievements)
- Publications, reports, published articles
- Documentation of awards/accomplishments
- Computer-related items
- Projects or group work completed/participated in

Education
- Course descriptions, module guides
- Assessments, test results, assignment feedback
- Awards
- Workshops, seminars, conferences attended
- Independent learning (things you've learned on your own or taught yourself)
- Certificates/evidence of special training

Personal activities
- Leadership positions held
- Hobbies or interests (time devoted to or photos)
- Participation in team sports
- Volunteer activities
- Organisations joined (all)
- Public speaking/presentations or performances
- Awards
- Travel

Personal qualities or strengths
- Strengths (personal qualities that will help you contribute to an employer or educational organisation)
- Teamwork and people skills, problem-solving, planning and organisation, time management, energy, discipline, motivation, persistence, responsibility, dependability, etc.
- Contributing to your family (teaching, caring for siblings, cooking – all require planning, responsibility, dependability)
- Helping your friends or working on extracurricular projects (may require teamwork, problem-solving skills, teaching skills, people skills)
- Raising a family and /or running a household (requires budgeting, organisation, time-management skills, adaptability)
- Keeping fit and healthy; being a member of a sports team (requires energy, discipline, motivation, persistence, teamwork)

The portfolio inventory can lull you into a false sense of security as you go away and collect all the awards, certificates, team photos you can find and put them in a large A4 folder, thinking that will constitute a portfolio. The key to portfolio development is the application of all the things on the inventory to your development.

You need to ask yourself the following questions for each piece of evidence you want to put in your portfolio:

- What existing experience and knowledge do I already have and can demonstrate for this piece of evidence?
- What are the implications for me, personally and professionally?
- What practical examples to demonstrate my skills and competence can I bring to this piece of evidence?
- What sources of information can I draw upon to inform this piece of evidence?
- What literary evidence can I provide to support this piece of evidence?
- How can I demonstrate best practice for this piece of evidence?
- What further development do I need to consider for this piece of evidence?

Not all the above questions will be appropriate for each piece of evidence but it should make you consider the reasons why you are submitting it. The reader of the portfolio needs to know why you have put a particular piece of evidence in the portfolio and what it demonstrates. This can be done by addressing the appropriate questions to items on the portfolio inventory or by providing triangulation of evidence. To do this you need to draw on three aspects of professional practice to support the evidence submitted to your portfolio. This model would be considered a reliable standard for any portfolio reflection/evidence (Fig. 3.1).

In practical terms:

1. You reflect on an experience, for example taken from a practice situation, and then draw on previous experiences in practice

2. You then consider the theory that has informed the experience or practice

3. Finally you support this with current literature or evidence-based practice tools.

By providing this triangulation of evidence you really demonstrate consideration of a wide range of resources, and it links all the essential qualities of professional practice.

The portfolio inventory provides evidence of personal development but the list of points does seem rather dry when considered in a health-care context. When you look at the inventory you need to consider each of the points in relation to interpersonal

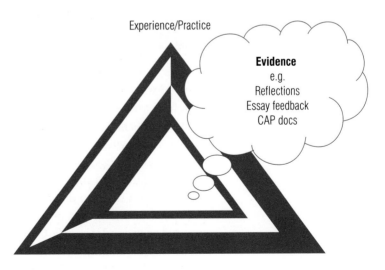

Figure 3.1 Triangulation of evidence

relationships and the context in which the care is given. This means the external environment and culture, your involvement in terms of health promotion, health maintenance and restoration, you as an advisor, counsellor and collaborator, the relationships, interactions and physical surroundings, and the perspective of the client (Walsh, 2000). These link to Goodman's levels of reflection and provide a range of external factors that should be influencing your practice.

Remember the triangulation of evidence of practice, theory and literature. The experience you have should be reflected on, bringing knowledge from previous practice, theory that has informed the experience and literature to support your reflection. All the elements of the triangulation of evidence can be linked to the external factors considered by Walsh (2000). You may look at the portfolio inventory now and feel overwhelmed in terms of how much evidence you need to provide, but remember, it is the quality of the evidence submitted, not the quantity, that is important. You do not need to submit a piece of evidence for everything on the portfolio inventory – you need to take a selection under each heading for which you can provide evidence.

Walsh (2000) states that what is important is not what is taught but what is learnt, not what message is sent but what is received, and this is what needs to come across in the portfolio. It is usually best to assimilate portfolio evidence on a running basis, as and when things happen. One of the aims of a portfolio is to stay focused on the quality of work by you the learner and the association of your work to the standards and goals of the professional or educational body.

Working with your portfolio

Chapter 2 looked at learning styles, and this can be very effective in terms of working with your portfolio and helping you to structure it. Hopefully you are feeling convinced of the added value of knowing your learning style – it may seem quite obvious now you have analysed how you learn best. Producing a portfolio is quite a methodical process and you need to be organised. If you are an Accommodator you may be feeling anxious at the thought of all the reflection you need to do and the fact you have to plan, catalogue and index all the pieces of work you put into the portfolio. If you are an Accommodator or a Converger you may prefer to have a 'ready-made' portfolio, as you will be given clear guidelines on how to structure and develop it. Once you have the structure organised it makes life much easier in terms of completing the portfolio (see the CD-ROM or Chapter 8).

Designing your portfolio

 When it comes to submitting or using your portfolio, consider that it presents you as a professional to an assessor, professional body or potential employer. It is essential that it portrays you in a professional manner. The CD-ROM portfolio with this book has templates for your CV and reflections that are presented professionally. The portfolio is a visual medium and you can add or create many different items to provide tangible proof of your activities or personal qualities. Having a visual representation of your skill will give you an opportunity to talk about why you have included a particular item and what it represents in terms of your abilities.

Arrange your portfolio in whichever way the assessor, professional body or potential employer requires it. If you have no guidelines you can organise your portfolio like your curriculum vitae or use the examples of portfolio structures in Chapter 8. A well-organised portfolio indicates that you are a serious candidate. If you prefer to keep a paper copy (and you may want to keep both a paper and electronic copy), presentation is very influential.

Key points | *Top tips*

- Buy the best quality cover that you can afford – it will last longer and look smarter.
- Inside your portfolio, use acetate or plastic sleeves to display and protect materials but do not be tempted to place too many sheets of paper in one sleeve – it can be irritating for the reader to constantly have to remove the papers to read.
- Include a table of contents to help direct the reader and use clear referencing if one piece of evidence informs one or more sections within your portfolio.
- Label and index materials, placing like materials together under a labelled tab so that you can turn to that section easily.

Using your portfolio

Your portfolio has a multitude of uses and it is a very important document. Its main function, when you begin to develop one, will depend on your position at the time. If you are a student it will be to pass the assessment and obtain your degree and professional qualification. If you are a qualified practitioner, it will be to satisfy your statutory body or professional requirements. Once you begin your portfolio development you will then start to see uses beyond the initial intention. Your portfolio should be used in conjunction with your application form to apply for a new job, it will inform your curriculum vitae and can guide your answers to the questions asked on the application form and in interview. Your portfolio can assist you in developing your personal development plan by identifying areas for development and indicating how you might best achieve your subsequent action plan through self-assessment and knowing your learning style. It can be used as part of an individual performance review or appraisal to support your development so far and plan future goals.

The portfolio should provide you with direction for your own development and learning. It should demonstrate how you are learning from practice or, if you feel you are not, it could help to make this evident so you can consider what action to take. It promotes reflective practice, therefore best practice. The portfolio is also a powerful tool for achieving accreditation by demonstrating prior learning. Most importantly it provides you with a picture of you and who you are as a practitioner as it combines all the elements of personal and professional learning.

Over to you

Imagine you are the head of a professional body, e.g. the Nursing and Midwifery Council. You have thousands of practitioners registered on your books who re-register every 3 years stating that they are competent and accountable practitioners. As the regulating council, you have to provide some assurance to the public that the professionals you represent are competent. How would you go about doing this? You have members on your books from diverse specialities, working at different levels. Manpower constraints make it impossible to set up systems under which all practitioners could actually be assessed every 3 years to ensure competence.

- Consider why a portfolio might address these issues.
- If you were assessing a portfolio, what would you be looking for it to include? (Bear in mind your responsibility to provide assurance that your members are competent and accountable.)

Many practitioners first become enthusiastic about portfolios when they realise their potential to create something unique about them and how they work. The possibilities are endless but it is often the fact there are so many possibilities that delays the starting of a portfolio. How do you create something that describes you and the way you work? There are so many different formats – which is the best one for you? These are frequently asked questions and there is

Consider why you bought this book.
What aspect of your portfolio development do you feel needs guidance?
   What do you think are the most important materials you need to start your portfolio?
   Always consider assessment at this stage, if the portfolio is being assessed it will be the biggest influencing factor as to what the contents of the portfolio are.
   Consider how you can collate the materials you need.

no definite answer. A portfolio is an individual piece of work and no two portfolios are produced or interpreted in the same way.

How can you demonstrate what you have learned?

Demonstrating what you have learned can often be considered the most difficult part of doing your portfolio. You can have lots of pieces of paper in your portfolio but how do they show your learning and consequent development? A ready-made portfolio can help you catalogue any documentation you have produced but you can run the risk of just having a collection of certificates, documents and papers. This does not constitute a portfolio – there has to be a personal element and evidence of growth and acquisition of skill. Redman (1994) claims that the essence of a portfolio is not experience, nor even what has been learned from that experience, it is the evidence of best practice.

The main experience students have of a portfolio seems to be the National Record of Achievements (Department for Education and Employment, 1991) or, more recently, the new Progress File (Department for Education and Skills, 2002), which can be valuable in terms of CV development, interview preparation and preparing you for considering the concept of a portfolio but does not come with guidelines on reflection and levels of reflection or with a requirement to be assessed.

I have interviewed a variety of newly qualified staff for staff nurse posts and asked to see their portfolios. I have been presented with a variety of folders, some excellent but the majority a disappointing catalogue of university module guides, continuous assessment of practice documents, certificates for basic life support (BLS) and moving and handling training records. While documents such as module guides and BLS certificates are useful to have in your portfolio, they need to be linked together, to demonstrate learning

Keywords

Synthesis
The combining of different
elements into a whole

and to provide evidence of best practice. A certificate to say that you have attended a study day may not provide an interviewer or professional body with evidence that you have actually learned anything from that study day if there is no proof of application and **synthesis**.

Reflective activity

It is always important to keep proof/certificates of mandatory training days and put these in your portfolio. You can enhance these by reflecting on occasions when you have used what you have learnt in practice.

As a health-care professional you will be trained in BLS. If you ever witness or participate in an emergency situation, you could reflect on the incident and relate it back to your BLS training. Was the training adequate? Did you feel able to help or did the situation seem overwhelming? If you did not participate yourself, did you witness another person going through BLS, looking at airway, breathing and circulation? If you were involved, could you ask someone to give you feedback on your performance?

You will be trained to move and handle patients correctly. Think back to your moving and handling training when you are working clinically. Are the techniques taught used in practice? If not, why do you think that is? Are you able to practise what you have learned?

These examples provide evidence of how you can use your training and how you can link your training to practice in the clinical area.

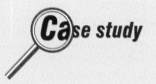 **Case study**

Helen's reflection

Helen is a newly qualified practitioner. She reflects:

When I qualified and took my first job I was petrified I'd get things wrong. I was worried I couldn't ask anyone for help or to show me what to do, especially in front of the patients and their relatives. I was wearing a uniform and badge that said I was qualified but, in reality, I felt anything but. After about 2 months I realised that the other members of the team did not expect me to perform like an 'old hand' and they were there to provide me with support. I also realised that patients and their relatives often just wanted somebody to discuss things with, regardless of my knowledge.

Reflective activity

How do you think Helen can reflect on this and demonstrate what she has learnt?
How can she provide evidence of good practice?

Making the most of your clinical experience for portfolio development

As a health-care professional, your training offers a rich source of experiences arising from the clinical aspects of your role, and this is an extremely important aspect of your portfolio. It is imperative that you get the most out of your clinical experience and your portfolio can help you to do this by identifying your learning needs. Your clinical practice will also inform your portfolio and the majority of reflective content within it. Planning before you go out on a clinical placement helps to identify what needs you have and what specific areas of your practice need to be developed. Your portfolio can assist in this process by having evidence at hand of your previous placement reports and skills inventories, which should be used to inform your future action plans. It also has information about how you learn and this can influence how you go about learning new skills on your placement.

Over to you

Ask yourself these questions before you go on a clinical placement (if you are already qualified, these questions can be asked of a new job or new role you may be considering):

1. What experiences do you think are available during this placement?
2. What aspects of your practice do you feel comfortable with?
3. What aspects of your practice need to be developed?
4. What preparations can you make to feel prepared for the placement? (e.g. reading, pre-placement visit, discussion with peers, university tutor support)

Adapted from the RCN Toolkit (Royal College of Nursing, 2002)

Try not to leave completing your portfolio until the last minute, even if you just scribble down notes after a shift or after a lecture that you found particularly interesting – this can be done during a coffee break. If you are too busy to do a 'proper' reflection, return to the notes later and reflect then. Often, hastily scribbled feelings experienced at the time of an incident are better revisited when you are away from the situation, to reflect objectively.

Reflection does not need to be time-consuming – indeed, a lack of time is a poor excuse for not thinking incidents and experiences over reflectively after they have occurred. It is not as though you will need to reflect in this way on everything that happens to you. But making reflection and portfolio development an inherent part of your practice will help you in developing your own knowledge and understanding for your practice. At the end of the day, it will probably save you time, because the learning achieved and the changes you make to your practice are immediate. Portfolio development should help us see the differences in health, social and psychological care experiences, so we can make informed decisions, recognising the strengths and weaknesses in our own experience.

If you feel at a complete loss as to how to start your portfolio, it is quite common to base it around your job description if you are qualified, or around your university guidelines and professional body competencies if you are a student. You can use the headings outlined in your job description or university guidelines and professional body competencies to form the headings for your portfolio. This provides you with a basic structure and can give you goals to work towards to ensure you are fulfilling your role. The list below, contains some examples of job description titles that are also relevant to prequalification practitioners and illustrates how you can incorporate them within your portfolio. This is covered in greater depth in Chapter 6.

Clinical responsibilities

- To deliver a high standard of individualised client care
    - Include reflections on practice that have made you consider the care you give, or give examples of evidence-based practice – how you changed your practice because of evidence from previous experience or literature/research
    - Include letters of thanks from clients (NB. Keep anonymous)
- To assess, plan, implement and evaluate care of patients from admission to discharge
    - Include a case history that you were involved with or, if you are currently a student, include essays discussing patient care
    - Write down details of a successful or unsuccessful discharge and reflect on how you felt about the process – consider what you have learnt from it.

Educational responsibilities

- To assist and participate in a teaching programme
    - If you are a student or newly qualified practitioner you may feel that you do not participate in teaching, but you do. It may not be as explicit as a formal teaching session, but providing information on a client's treatment to clients and relatives can be considered as teaching, especially if you check their knowledge and ensure they have understood what you have told them. For example, when preparing a patient for theatre, you inform them of what to expect postoperatively so they are prepared.

– Sharing experiences is a good example of informal teaching of peers – you may have experience of caring for a client with a certain condition whereas a fellow student/member of staff does not, and you can share this information with them.

This approach to portfolio planning is acceptable but you may find that basing your portfolio on your job description directs you into very specific areas. When you want a promotion or career change, your portfolio is quite restricted, and may not demonstrate all round growth or development and the diversity you might need for a career change. A more individual way of structuring your portfolio is to base it on your learning style inventory. By using your learning style inventory you produce a portfolio that addresses your needs, your strengths and weaknesses. You can highlight areas in which you need to improve and you can then give specific details of how you have gone about gaining that experience.

Reflective activity

Think of the main themes in your professional life. There will be some cross-over and different areas covered but what are the quintessential elements that make up your job (e.g. client care, education, professional development)? Can they be used as section headings for your portfolio? Consider whether this approach would accurately reflect your development.

Benefits of reflection and portfolio development to your practice

Chapter 2 discussed how to link theory to practice through experiential learning, reflection and portfolio development. Within these connections it is important to consider why the linking of theory to practice is important. The essence of caring and wanting to develop yourself and your practice is to improve client care and provide best practice. This should be apparent in your portfolio entries. There needs to be a clear reason as to why you have included the evidence you have, in terms of:

● Benefit to clients and their carers

● Benefit to you as a developing practitioner

● Benefit to the wider organisation.

Consider the following Case study concerning Beatriz.

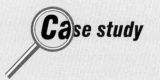

Case study

Beatriz's communication

Beatriz was an overseas student and reflected on an experience she had while feeding an elderly client. During the process she spoke quietly to herself in her native language, asking why she was feeding the client when the client clearly did not want feeding. Beatriz heard a voice behind ask in her native tongue, 'Well, why are you?' Unknown to her, the client in the next bed could speak Beatriz's language.

There are several issues raised here but the one Beatriz predominantly wanted to focus on was the fact that feeding clients is considered an essential part of nursing care. It is important that clients receive adequate nutrition, and there is little room to argue on this point, but the client clearly did not want to be fed. Beatriz had done her 'duty' but, while feeding the client, was questioning what she was doing. On reflection, she wished she had taken that questioning one step further and considered what the client felt was good for them. The conclusion to the reflection was that when the client was due to have the next meal, Beatriz would consider alternatives such as dietary supplements instead of persuading the client to eat food she did not want or feel up to eating.

This may seem a simple solution, and it is, but it can be something as simple as seeing what is good for the client that transforms their experience of illness and alters the way in which you think as a health-care professional. What you may feel is right or what you are taught is the right thing to do may not fit in with how the client thinks. Beatriz changed her perspective and enhanced client care by thinking about what the client wanted rather than what she had been taught and told do to. The future of health care lies in the flexibility and individualised care offered to clients.

RRRRRRapid recap

Check your progress so far by working through each of the following questions.

1. What key questions should you consider each time you want to put a piece of evidence into your portfolio?
2. List five things you have to remember in order to produce a well-organised paper portfolio.

If you have difficulty with either of the questions, read through the section again to refresh your understanding before moving on.

References

Department for Education and Employment (1991) *National Records of Achievement*. DfEE, London.

Department for Education and Skills (2002) *Progress File*. DfES, London.

Redman, W. (1994) *Portfolios for Development*. Kogan Page, London.

Royal College of Nursing (2002) *Helping Students Get the Best from their Practice Placements: An RCN toolkit*. RCN, London.

Walsh, M. (2000) *Nursing Frontiers: Accountability and the boundaries of care*. Butterworth-Heinemann, Oxford.

4

Portfolio as assessment

Herman Wheeler

Learning outcomes

By the end of this chapter you should be able to:

- Explain the concept of assessment and distinguish between formative and summative assessment of portfolios and profiles

- Distinguish between a portfolio and a profile in terms of definition and assessment

- Identify what assessors are looking for when marking and judging portfolios

- Take a learning outcome from your study programme and analyse it in terms of what portfolio evidence could demonstrate your understanding and achievement of it

- Identify pieces of evidence that may be used to support claims of personal learning and development

- Highlight and justify the importance of considering the structure and presentation of a portfolio

'Portfolio as assessment' is a very broad subject indeed. For example, one could look at it in terms of:

- A portfolio-based assignment as one of the assessment items within a portfolio of assessment for a given programme of study or a module

- A course of study or continuous professional development programme actually making the development of a 'whole' portfolio the assessment requirement for that programme/course of study

- The need to address the question, 'How can we use a portfolio to assess whether students have achieved the learning outcomes of a module or programme of study?' Indeed, how can the student use a portfolio to assess personal development needs?

- Is it really possible to assess a portfolio?

The last question could lead to two further logical and related ones; firstly, how do we assess portfolios? Secondly, who may assess a portfolio?

One could also reflect on the notion of you assessing whether the portfolio you have developed (or are currently developing) was actually fulfilling some previously stated criteria related to personal, academic and professional growth. Could the section offer you the opportunity to develop competence to decide your own criteria of what constitutes 'good', 'bad', 'not so good', outright 'poor' portfolios, as the case might be? As a student you and others (e.g. teachers, lecturers and other course providers) can use your portfolio to decide whether you have developed academically, personally and professionally. Monitoring criteria can be particularly useful for this.

Students and qualified staff also need to be able to ascertain how 'significant others' might judge them through their portfolios. 'Significant others' in the present context include lecturers and personal tutors, professional and course validating bodies, external examiners, clinical supervisors, mentors, assessors, peers and

- Explain how the notions of academic credit values, academic levels, APL, APEL, National Credit Accumulation and Transfer Schemes, pre- and postregistration education and practice development and life-long learning relate to the notion of portfolio assessment.

candidate selectors for advanced continuing professional development programmes, potential employers, employers, managers and other stakeholders.

Finally, academic staff (who may well not have compiled a portfolio as part of their own training) are often required to guide their personal tutees in portfolio development. They also have to assist with assessing students' portfolios and sometimes require guidance on how to do this.

This chapter therefore touches upon all the above-mentioned issues. However, although the approach taken is introductory, rather than deep, and is therefore geared towards preregistration health-care students, the chapter should also prove helpful to more senior health-care practitioners. It goes without saying that the experienced and skilled practitioner still needs, at times, to revisit fundamental concepts to aid critical reflection *in* and *on* practice. This is seen as one of the ways of updating oneself in order to enhance standards in professional practice. If you are a more experienced health-care practitioner, you should find the chapter a useful revision at least. Moreover, you may in fact be a mentor, assessor and supervisor of preregistration health-care students and as such you may sometimes find yourself involved in guiding students in portfolio development. You may also help with health-care curriculum development and with teaching and assessing the progress of students, in which case you should also find the chapter helpful.

An obvious and fundamental first step is to pose the question: What is assessment? What do we mean by assessment and can portfolios and profiles be assessed?

In order to answer both questions it is necessary to ask: 'What does "assessment" mean?' In assessing something we are bringing critical judgement to bear upon it. It could be knowledge, skills, competencies or attitudes. It may be an essay written by someone, a speech or other type of verbal presentation. It may be a clinical activity such as giving medication to a patient, dressing, washing or feeding a patient. It could be the assessment of skills or competencies that someone claims to possess. It could be the assessment of attitudes, in spite of their relative difficulty to assess. We may be judging the quality of our own or someone else's work. We may be assessing or judging a portfolio or a profile drawn from a portfolio. We are making decisions about what is good and commendable about the portfolio or profile and what is not good about it. We may be judging someone's competencies for a given role, for example an ability to lead a group. We are bringing critical assessment and evaluative judgement to decide what is good, bad or indifferent about the person, situation or thing. Judging or assessing portfolios enables us to determine students' achievements and competencies.

Historical perspective

As discussed in Chapter 1, portfolio development and assessment were 'adopted' from fine arts, where portfolios are used to display an artist's work in terms of depth, breadth, interest and abilities (Jongsma, 1989; Moya and O'Malley, 1994). Within health-care education and practice, portfolio and profile development and assessment are moving fast. Portfolio assessment is an acceptable alternative to conventional assessments and 'standardised testing' (Flood and Lapp, 1989; Valencia, 1990a, b). Moreover standardised testing is seen as **antithetical** to *process* learning (Moya and O'Malley, 1994), which promotes process-driven student outcomes over product-driven learning outcomes and objectives. From anecdotal feedback received from my undergraduate nursing and physiotherapy students, who have been exposed to both product- and process-driven learning and assessment methods, there is some evidence to support the premise that portfolio development, as a process-driven option, promotes 'deep', as opposed to 'surface', learning (Biggs, 1979, 1999; Tiwari and Tang, 2003). I would argue, however, that there is a need for portfolio development and assessment to focus on both the product produced by the student and the process that the students describe as enabling them to produce it.

In the School of Health Sciences where I work, the concept of portfolio development by students was first introduced in 1995 for health-care students undertaking a post-experienced diploma/masters programme. In developing their portfolios for summative assessment, as part-fulfilment of the assessment requirements for the course, the students had a lot of choice over the contents of their portfolios. Central to their choice of portfolio content was the fact that they had to develop it to address their personal and professional development needs, relating where appropriate to learning outcomes within the Professional Development module. Additionally, students on the clinical route of this programme had to address in their portfolio the now defunct English National Board for Nursing, Midwifery and Health Visiting 10 Characteristics for a Higher Award Framework.

In 1996, portfolio development was introduced into the undergraduate nursing programme, although the assessment linked

Keywords

Antithetical
Directly opposite or contrasting

to this was strictly formative. The concept of portfolio was introduced to these students through lectures, workshops and informal one-to-one sessions with personal tutors and with lecturers linked to the Professional Development module, but mainly at the request of the student. Students were encouraged to start the process of developing a portfolio, which they would then be able to continue to develop when they qualified. It was a steep learning and development curve for both the students and the academic staff. Many staff had not hitherto developed their own personal portfolio or even written a reflective piece for a portfolio or a personal journal, let alone supporting and confidently advising students on the development of their own.

Some students found the initiative attractive and interesting, some did not. Personal tutors had to increase their understanding of the notion of portfolio and portfolio building speedily to be available to offer students helpful advice and support. Indeed, students were encouraged to call upon their personal tutors for help in developing their portfolios. At this time the notion of reflection and reflective practice, life-long learning and the keeping of a personal learning journal were being emphasised within the undergraduate curriculum; this strengthened and supported the notion of portfolio building.

Students entering the undergraduate nursing programme in the 1997–98 academic year were required to submit small pieces of personal reflections from their personal learning journals for formative assessment only. They received written feedback on these and were advised to include these reflective pieces in their developing portfolio.

In 1999, with the introduction of a new undergraduate curriculum, portfolio development took on greater emphasis within the curriculum and all new students entering the degree programme were required to develop their portfolio from the first week of the course. Portfolio-building workshops, formal and informal teaching and support were initiated and students were provided with a portfolio framework document. Assessment of portfolio work now became a formative as well as a summative exercise and for the first time the assessment also included the assessment of the whole portfolio in the final year of the course. The portfolio assessment entity developed incrementally. In years 1, 2 and 3 students had to hand in a short written reflective piece from their journal for summative assessment under the Professional Development module assessment requirements. Formal and informal workshops, lectures and individual guidance sessions on portfolio building were provided

Keywords

Aegis
Patronage

to the students and formalised under the **aegis** of the Professional Development module. In spring 2003 the 1999 cohort of undergraduates will be required to submit, for the first time, their entire portfolio document for summative assessment. This will form 100% of the assessment weighting for this module.

Portfolio assessment must not be seen purely in terms of how others judge the student's developed or developing portfolio (and through this the student personally, academically and professionally). Portfolio assessment must also be seen in terms of what Moya and O'Malley (1994) describe as the portfolio developer's *planning*, *collection* and *analysis* of the data contained in the portfolio. In other words, portfolio assessment is also about how students themselves set about planning the portfolio, deciding critically what they collect to go into it and the analytical processes they select and apply to the portfolio data collected. Yet, curiously, in the general education context it appears that guidelines for portfolio development and assessment are few (Moya and O'Malley, 1994).

It seems fair to state therefore that more portfolio development and assessment guidelines are needed to support the pedagogical 'shift' from teacher-centred teaching and learning to student-centred learning that portfolio development and problem-based learning so strongly support.

Claims we make in assessing portfolios

If we are judging or assessing someone's portfolio we are, by implication, claiming to have the capacity and capability to make a valid judgement about the quality of that portfolio. Moreover, we are judging people's skills, knowledge and attitudes by the evidence they put in their portfolios. With respect to the portfolio itself, we may perhaps focus on the skill with which it has been put together, the clarity it conveys in demonstrating to the reader how the compiler has developed, whether evidence for claims made is clear and appropriate and so on. This implies that we have some predetermined criteria of what constitutes good standard of performance in portfolio development. Is the portfolio good, not so good, poor, etc?

Can we speak in such simplistic terms, though? As the development of this chapter will show, judging portfolios is not the easiest of tasks and it could be inappropriate to use such extreme value labels as 'good', 'bad' or 'poor' to describe a portfolio. There are a number of reasons for this: first is the individual nature of this personal and professional developmental and learning tool. Secondly, a portfolio, being such a private and individual compilation, actually charts its owner's personal and professional development. It charts new skills, competencies, new knowledge and understanding, all judged perhaps against predetermined goals and criteria, set by the portfolio writer/developer and other stakeholders.

It is often the case that in health-care education and training programmes your learning outcomes are predetermined, i.e. laid down by the course directives. For example, there are specific modular learning outcomes that you must attain in order to be credited with the course or specific modules. This is not to say that you are denied latitude, autonomy and individual decision-making opportunities in terms of choice of specific developmental objectives, within the framework of course-determined learning outcomes. Learning outcomes that are aimed at developing self-awareness, information processing, critical reflection, decision-making, interpersonal communication skills, empathy for others, problem solving, and so on, are themselves sufficiently broad and flexible to provide you with latitude and freedom for some choice within wider predetermined objectives.

In other words, predetermined programme objectives for portfolio building need to recognise your need for some degree of self-determination regarding personal development needs. Put frankly, if you are developing a portfolio you need the freedom to work out your own development needs, even if some of these must of necessity address predetermined course outcomes. In assessing students' portfolios, therefore, assessors must be careful to take on board students' own perceptions of their needs and aspirations.

It is clear that, unless the assessor or portfolio-marking panel can answer the questions in the box on the next page, they are unlikely to be doing a good job at assessing students' portfolios rigorously and objectively. After all, a portfolio is not an independent entity with a life of its own. It exists because somebody has put it together. It is meant to demonstrate, with clear evidence, the portfolio builder's personal and professional development needs (including knowledge and understanding, skills and competencies, as well as any other attributes considered appropriate) and an analysis of how these needs were met.

Some important questions portfolio assessors need to ask themselves prior to assessing and marking students portfolios:

● Are there specific module/programme/course-related portfolio development criteria against which this portfolio was developed and against which it should be assessed?

● Have I taken into account the portfolio developer's own individualistic portfolio development criteria, balanced against module/programme/course-determined portfolio development requirements, including specific learning outcomes?

● Has the student who developed this portfolio indicated any special considerations s/he would like taken into account when this portfolio is being judged?

● Has the portfolio developer set out for the attention of the marker/assessor/portfolio-assessment panel any special self-acknowledged limitations experienced in the process of the portfolio development and/or in the final portfolio product?

● In developing the portfolio, what did the student identify as his/her personal and professional development and learning needs?

● What specific skills, competencies, forms of knowledge and attitudes did the student set out to achieve within the context of self-development through portfolio building?

Formative and summative assessment and their relationship to portfolio assessment

○┅ᴛ *Keywords*
....

Formative
An informal assessment where the marks do not count towards your final result

Summative
A formal assessment where the marks count towards the module or diploma/degree final result

In the educational context, particularly in health-care curriculum planning, delivery and evaluation, we often talk about **formative** and **summative** assessment. Either type of assessment could be used in the context of assessing portfolios and profiles.

To assess something formatively usually means that a set of results will not normally be used to decide that a student has failed or passed a module or programme of study. Formative results may be more important than simply deciding pass or fail. For instance, formative assessments may be undertaken early in a module or programme of study in order to provide you with essential diagnostic feedback relating to performance, strengths and weaknesses and what needs to be done to correct weaknesses and build upon strengths. Weaknesses need to be addressed in order to avoid failure in subsequent summative assessments, since summative assessments can decide pass or fail and therefore whether you remain on a course. The summative assessment can decide whether you are awarded your degree or diploma, or whether you have failed.

Top tips

- Do not take a formative assessment of your portfolio, or any other piece of work for that matter, for granted.

In the case of a portfolio, a formative assessment in years 1 and 2 of a 3-year programme, for example, may not only help to provide you with feedback on how you are progressing in these early years (formative assessment) but may serve to inform the final summative portfolio assessment grade in the final year. This shows how what appears to some students, early on in a course, to be 'just a formative assessment' can turn out to be most critical. Formative assessment results can be of immense value to you in the here and now and in the future also. Later, we will discuss the importance of professional portfolios to you as a health-care practitioner throughout your career.

Applying the concept of formative and summative assessment of portfolio to the reality of a healthcare degree or diploma programme, the following picture emerges. In years 1 and 2 you could be assessed both formatively and summatively in portfolio development. For your summative assessment you might be asked to undertake portfolio-based reflective assignments that you must pass. Or you might be asked to draw on your portfolio to reflect on and demonstrate your learning with evidence in relation to a number of module-related learning outcomes.

Introduction to portfolio building should be undertaken early on in year 1 and this portfolio-building process should continue throughout the course. The bonus of continuous formative assessment is that it provides and guides the development of your portfolio. If your portfolio is submitted for summative assessment at the end of your course, it will be ready for formal assessment.

The formative assessment of your developing portfolio takes a more informal approach. You have the opportunity to discuss the development of your portfolio with, for example, your personal tutor, a lecturer of your choice, the facilitator of your problem-based learning group, your peers and/or any other person you choose. You can, if you wish, submit your developing portfolio for critical scrutiny in an appropriate problem-based learning session. Feedback will be provided. You should use such opportunities to confirm your strengths as well as to identify your weaknesses in portfolio development.

To facilitate such a process a non-threatening atmosphere needs to be promoted. It enables you to assess your performance through open discussion with other people. A sensitive and sensible student will use constructive feedback to modify and improve performance, whether in portfolio development or in some other skill.

Over to you

Identify what you would expect to gain from submitting your developing portfolio for critique to a small group of your peers and/or your lecturer or personal tutor.

Identify the sort of questions you expect the small group of your peers and/or your lecturer/personal tutor to put to you before they begin to assess your portfolio.

Using the framework below, note each gain that you might expect from this exercise. For each gain suggest possible forms of evidence that you could use to demonstrate your learning/development/gain. Draw a larger version of the table if necessary.

Learning/development/gain	Possible forms of evidence
a)	
b)	
c)	
d)	

Key points   Top tips

- To assess is to make critical judgement about the worth of something; put simply, is the thing/situation or event 'good' or 'bad'?

- Assessment can be *formative* (diagnostic and helpful to the student), or it can be *summative*, i.e. making final decisions as to success or failure.

- A portfolio may be assessed formatively or summatively.

- There are important questions that portfolio assessors need to ask themselves before they start to judge a student's portfolio.

- Other people, e.g. peers, teachers, may help you to progress the development of your portfolio through scrutiny, linked to your own prior set criteria, among others, and from the informal feedback provided.

- Both formative and summative assessment can be crucial to the student being assessed. Therefore in portfolio development neither assessment should be taken for granted by the student/portfolio builder.

- Judging portfolios may not be simply a question of using extreme value terms such as 'good' or 'bad' portfolios, as portfolios are individually developed learning and development tools and will require application of objective and subjective reasoning.

Assessment of portfolio or profile: the private and public perspective

If you are to be assessed via a portfolio of evidence of your development (in terms of, for example, knowledge and understanding, competencies, attitudes, continued proactive readiness to learn and to serve) what should you present for public examination? You may not wish to submit the entire portfolio for public scrutiny because, at this stage, it contains some materials that you do not wish to share with a public audience. On the other hand, you may have developed your portfolio with the exact intention of presenting it in its entirety for public gaze.

It all depends on the specific purpose for developing the portfolio. If you clearly intended to have the entire portfolio content examined, then from the outset you may have chosen to include only evidence that you feel comfortable to share with others. There is also the question of what is considered ethical to disclose.

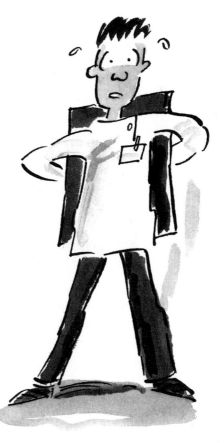

Decide what is for public viewing in your portfolio and what is to be kept private

Key points Top tips

- This is where the distinction between a profile and a portfolio is made. A profile is drawn from the portfolio and is meant to contain those pieces of evidence of our development that we wish to put up for public scrutiny, examination or assessment, depending on the audience.

In the situation where the portfolio's owner is applying for a job, s/he may just wish to use the portfolio to develop a curriculum vitae. In this case, depending on what you consider those who advertise the job are looking for, you select those pieces of portfolio evidence that enable you to present the best image of yourself to impress those who are going to examine your CV for the job. On the other hand, you may decide to take the entire portfolio to the interview.

Many candidates who attend interviews for a place on an undergraduate nursing programme bring with them what they call their 'record of achievement' (National Record of Achievement; Department for Education and Employment, 1991) or, more currently, the new Progress File (Department for Education and Skills, 2002). This is similar to a profile but obviously not as highly or as fully developed as the profile extracted from a personal and professional portfolio. So these candidates are already used to the idea of selecting from their repertoire of achievements those elements they think are likely to show them off in the best light. This activity of putting together a 'record of achievement' document is good preparation for extracting effective and impressive material evidence from a portfolio.

Addressing a learning outcome in the context of a portfolio-based assignment

Earlier in this chapter we looked at health-care students who have been asked to undertake a portfolio-based assignment. Since they are being asked to select evidence from their portfolio to demonstrate their learning and understanding, new skills and competencies, in respect to a given number of module learning outcomes, they are clearly not expected within the course to present their entire portfolio for assessment. They are being asked to structure their presentation in such a way as to show their critical reflection and understanding of each learning outcome. In the process they are expected to use relevant evidence from their portfolio to support what it is they are claiming in terms of new skills, competencies, knowledge and understanding. The evidence must focus on the learning outcome(s) being addressed.

The structured work, containing relevant pieces of portfolio evidence, is the public profile in this case. It must relate and explain understanding of the specific learning outcome being addressed. The work presented for public scrutiny in relation to the learning outcome(s) could address, for example, issues and questions such as:

- What does this learning outcome mean? Evidence of my understanding of the meaning?

- What is my understanding of the implications of this learning outcome? For me personally? Professionally? For my learning and development? For my interactions?

- What practical examples, scenarios, experiences and situations can I draw on to demonstrate my learning, my knowledge and understanding in relation to this particular learning outcome?

- What information source from the classroom (e.g. critical discussions, notes, workshop activities and discoveries, handouts, lectures, experiential learning examples) can I draw on and present as evidence?

- What pre-university and university experiences (including classroom and social experiences) have I reflected on and noted in my portfolio that I can now draw on and use as supporting evidence?

- What clinical experiences, situations, scenarios, interactions can I draw on that will help me demonstrate my learning and understanding in relation to this learning outcome?

- What literature evidence can I use to support my reflection and critical evaluation of the issues that surface when I examine my new learning, skills, attitudes and competencies?

- What theoretical, ethical, legal, clinical practice issues and implications are involved? What evidence have I got for these claims? What references are appropriate to back up my views?

- What reflections have I made in the past and noted in my portfolio that I can now draw on to support the claims I am now making about my understanding, knowledge and professional growth in relation to this learning outcome?

- How do I further develop my knowledge, skills and attitudes in relation to this specified learning outcome, as well as others that have emanated from my reflection on the first learning outcome?
- In my reflection on the specified learning outcome, have I addressed the issues of my knowledge, skills and competencies, feelings, attitudes and future directions in terms of my action theory for further learning and development?

Over to you

As an example of a portfolio-based reflective assignment, consider you have been asked to: 'Provide evidence to demonstrate your learning and understanding of the use of self assessment and portfolio in the management of learning'.

Making some assumptions about what the marker/assessor/examiner might be looking for, how would you approach this question?

Use the framework on the next page to sketch the approach you would take.

Possible approaches to take: Important considerations	Development actions and evidence

Table 4.1 is an example of a detailed and comprehensive plan for the portfolio-based reflective question in the above Over to you box. Compare it with your answer.

Table 4.1 Sample plan for portfolio-based reflective assignment

Possible approaches to take: Important considerations	Developmental actions and evidence
• Remember: *'portfolio-based'* work	Clear plan, structure
• **Evidence** (Portfolio? Others? Pre-university? University? Clinical practice? Social? Family? Business interaction? Literature? School? Work? Church? Play? Personal experience? Other people's experience?)	Descriptions, critical discussion, reflection, relevant evidence; examples?
	Relevant portfolio reflective evidence?
• As this is a PD module, emphasis is on growth and development through understanding of *'self assessment'* & *'use of portfolio'* to *manage* learning	Other relevant evidence?
	Meaning of self-assessment? (own knowledge, ideas, experiences, examples?)
• Self-assessment?	Literature: on 'self-assessment' & 'portfolio'? (references, quotes, etc., use texts books, internet sources, journals, classroom, work group, notes, lectures, PBL sessions, other sources/publications)
• Portfolio linked to managing learning?	
• What's *learning* anyway?	
• *Manage learning* (learning as development – personal, academic and professional)	Portfolio evidence/reflection re *self-assessment* in relation to *management of learning*
• How can 'self assessment' inform management of learning? Cite examples	My learning? Learning in general?
	What is learning? Link to self assessment, portfolio
• How can 'portfolio development' inform management of learning? Cite examples	How can self-assessment inform learning? One's ability to learn? Any person's ability to learn?
• What is self-assessment? How does this inform management of learning? Examples?	Have I assessed myself? How? (evidence?)
• What is a portfolio & how does portfolio inform management of learning? Examples?	Who am I really? (evidence?); self awareness
• Remember critical reflection. Word limit?*	My learning style? Personal/cognitive style? (evidence?)
• Remember supporting references, within text & final reference list*	Preferred learning style, techniques and strategies used? Results?
• What evidence goes into the text?	Reflect on different ways to self-assess? (e.g. questionnaires, l/style inventories, personality tests, self-examination; feedback from peers, teachers, patients, mentors, clinical supervisors, essays, exams & portfolio assessment, etc.)
• Remember your appendices, all cross-referenced with text*	
• Any other assignment criteria not addressed?*	Usefulness of knowing strengths & weaknesses – evidence?
	Use & implications of knowing self in managing learning? Implications of strengths, weaknesses?
	Usefulness of portfolios in managing learning?

* Can be moved here from the left-hand column

A list of examples of portfolio materials that you can submit as evidence of development, skills, knowledge, competencies and achievement is given in Chapter 3.

Key points Top tips

- Portfolios are a collection of evidence to demonstrate personal and professional development, knowledge, skills, attitudes, other achievements.

- Portfolios are usually private to the compiler but can be made public in whole or in part through focused extractions to produce 'public' profiles of attainment and potential serving capabilities. These 'public' profiles may be useful to support one's CV.

- The focus and purpose of the profile, influenced by personal and ethical considerations, should dictate what goes into a profile for public gaze.

- Assessment of a person's (e.g. a student's) competencies, skills, knowledge and attitudes may be assessed via their entire portfolio or by way of a profile extracted from the portfolio.

- In a module of study it is possible to test students' achievement of learning outcomes through entire portfolios or portfolio-based reflective assignments, including reflective journals. (See the Over to you exercise and Table 4.1.)

- Portfolio and profile materials and pieces of evidence to support learning, development and achievement of skills, knowledge and competencies can be varied.

Versatility of portfolio and profile development and assessment across professions

Currently, portfolio development and assessment as proof of personal, academic and professional growth, together with possession of potentially useful and much needed skills and competencies are not an exclusive province of the caring professions. While it is true that currently doctors, nurses, physiotherapists, podiatrists, social workers and psychologists (among others) are having to develop portfolios as evidence of professional development, these are not the only professions that have discovered the usefulness of portfolio building. Indeed, you may already have experienced the pride associated with carrying your art, engineering drawings, woodwork and craft portfolios to and from school. How proud you were to show these off to parents, friends and potential employers! In doing so you were probably thinking, 'Just look at my achievements!' 'See what I can do!' See what I will be able to do if you employ me in your company!'

If we think about it, what better way for artists to show off their artistic profile to potential users of their skills and competencies? We may ask, 'Did you really draw these?' We may just say, 'Wow! Brilliant!' We are actually assessing the artist's potential to produce an excellent portrait of us for that prominent place on our living room wall. Here, then, the artist's portfolio has given us an opportunity to assess and evaluate his/her actual and potential skill to do a good job of work for us. Artists have always been inclined to walk about with their portfolio of drawings and paintings. So while portfolio development and the assessment of skills, competencies and talents may be relatively new to the health-care professions, it is an established method of showing off skills, talents and competencies in the fields of fine arts and architecture.

I recall one occasion when I was studying to qualify as a lawyer. A number of doctors, architects and surveyors, among other professionals, were on the same postgraduate course. So one day I asked a particular architect how credible he considered himself as an architect. I really wanted to find out if he was good enough to be asked to undertake the drawings for a house extension I was planning. Realising what my motives were, the guy replied, 'Not only am I a qualified and experienced architect, I also hold chartered status, run my own company and have several architectural designs under my belt. Would you like to see my portfolio?' Before I could answer, he added, 'On second thoughts, I don't think I have my entire portfolio in the car. However I have a small but appropriate profile of my work. Would you like to see it?' Having seen his professional profile, I was so impressed with the quality of his work that I asked him straight away to do my drawings.

The point is that this architect not only had his profile ready to show to a potential client, he was also able to produce, at a later date, a comprehensive portfolio of his work. So artists and architects have always realised the value of portfolios and their skills and talents are often judged by the quality of their profile and portfolio.

Key points Top tips

- Portfolios and profiles are used in a variety of professions.
- Artists and architects have always used portfolios and profiles to demonstrate their skills and abilities.
- Compared to artists and architects, health-care professionals are relative newcomers in the development and use of portfolios and profiles.
- A well put together portfolio/profile can be a good seller of its compiler's skills.

Structure and organisation of a portfolio for assessment

Portfolio size and structure/layout

Students who are required to present whole portfolios for assessments often ask, 'How big should my portfolio be?' 'Is there a word limit?' These are difficult questions to answer and a valid answer depends on so many things. One of the most important criteria that portfolio assessors look for is the actual structure, organisation and overall quality of presentation of the portfolio. The early pages, introduction and contents pages are crucial in terms of explaining clearly how the portfolio is organised, giving a description of sections and subsections of the portfolio and where to locate specific pieces of evidence. What can be found and where are important to the marker/assessor. A clear, organised and intelligible layout will always put the assessor in a good frame of mind for assessing the entire work.

It is difficult to put a word limit on a portfolio for assessment for a number of reasons. It is personal to its compiler. Which areas of personal and professional development to concentrate on and submit for public scrutiny and assessment is a matter for personal consideration by you, the compiler. The areas chosen will be dictated by your original self-assessment and evaluation of personal and professional development needs, your intentions and what you consider relevant and important. Also, you will have to consider what will fit and inform the contexts and the objectives of the situation and the exercise.

> **Key points** | **Top tips**
>
> ● A very thick portfolio that appears in two or three volumes may not necessarily be the most impressive and high-quality presentation. Quality is what matters and clear explanations of what? why? evidence? where?

That is not to say that a very thick portfolio, or even a portfolio delivered in more than one volume, is not a good portfolio. Indeed, I have seen some very good, some not so good and some poor portfolios presented in a very thick single volume and in multivolume formats also. Equally, I have seen some impressive, some not so impressive and some poor portfolio presentations in slim single volumes.

Top tips

- Good portfolios are usually well explained in terms of what they contain, where the materials are located and how to locate particular pieces of evidence for claims being made. It is usually necessary to cross reference one relevant part or section of a portfolio with another to enhance clarity of presentation.

Inclusion/exclusion issues and other structure characteristics

There must be a reason for including materials in the portfolio. What is the reason? Explain why things are included in the portfolio. Do not just throw things in without explaining why they are there. If you decide to divide your portfolio into sections or chapters, what is each section/chapter about? Use clear descriptive headings. While you may want to include all your work in the portfolio, you must be selective. Develop a screening procedure to exclude irrelevance, etc.

Relevance and comprehensiveness matter and are part of the quality of your portfolio. These qualities relate to your capability in terms of depth and breadth of development, quality of portfolio data collection and analysis, formal and informal assessment of the capabilities and attainment you are claiming, process and product learning dimensions, learning and achievement in the linguistic, cognitive, psychomotor, affective and attitudinal domains, and teacher- and student-derived learning outcomes. Comprehensiveness also addresses both academic and professional (including theoretical and clinical) development issues.

Moya and O'Malley (1994) suggest the need for 'predetermined and systematic' planning, which must address issues such as the purpose and content of the portfolio, data collection and student performance criteria, as well as the expectations of teachers and other significant stakeholders.

Your contents page will help define your structure. In addition to the suggested hierarchy of headings given in Chapter 3, it may be that you wish to begin your portfolio with the following:

- Who you are
- Title page or overall description of what the work/presentation is about
- Introduction, including description of how the portfolio is organised, where to find content/evidence, etc. Make clear what personal and professional developments you are submitting/claiming, what the evidence is for these and where to locate it.

These divisions are obviously somewhat artificial but are recommended because they lead to a neat, highly structured portfolio presentation. Indeed, analysis of personal and professional development issues under prescribed sections of the portfolio document may well show that content in one section overlaps that in another.

Key points **Top tips**

Good portfolios:
- Carefully address identified personal and professional development needs
- Show the initial level and amount of those needs
- Show the strategies identified and developed to realise the needs
- Articulate how the needs were achieved
- Articulate the present level of attainment of those needs in terms of knowledge, skills and attitudes.

Key points Top tips

- A good portfolio is also futuristic in its outlook. It shows your future intentions regarding further development of your needs, as well as related ones spun off from the originally identified needs.
- Moreover, such a portfolio will give an indication of your intentions and proposed strategies to achieve the remaining and/or new needs. You are meant to be descriptive, critically reflective, analytical, realistic and discerning to present a good portfolio. Analysing personal development must centre on the past, the present and the future.

Materials and evidence

Evidence must be clearly set out, and must reflect clearly the personal development under discussion. It may be possible for one piece of evidence to inform more than one learning outcome or personal development issue. If this is so it must be clearly pointed out to the reader or assessor. The portfolio inventory in Chapter 3 provides examples of the sort of portfolio materials and therefore evidence that may be used to inform claims being made. A critical reflection that first describes, then analyses the issues uncovered in the examination of an experience, together with an explanation of how emerging theories have been skilfully applied to one's learning and development are key tactics to use in your portfolio. Do not be afraid to empower yourself, in valuing your own views, feelings, knowledge and understanding of the situation. However, back up critical personal analysis and evaluation with reference to literature, practical examples and, where appropriate, evidence arising from discussions with other people who can substantiate any claims you make.

Specified learning outcomes should be addressed

Good portfolios will, where appropriate, address any specific learning outcomes that you have been asked to address. For example, if you are told that in developing your portfolio you must, among other things, address certain learning outcomes, then make sure you have done so. There is not much point in concentrating purely on the issues of development that grab your fancy and ignoring specific areas and objectives that you are expected to address in developing your portfolio.

Student autonomy

Assessors will be looking to see that, as well as areas that you have chosen yourself for personal development, you have also addressed specific objectives and learning outcomes set by the assessors. You should study any specific portfolio development guidelines and marking criteria given by assessors. Note, however, that educators who ask you to develop portfolios for module and programme assessment, whether in whole or in part, will be aware that a portfolio is very personal thing that gives you latitude and empowerment. Educators therefore value flexibility and student autonomy.

However, you must not forget that, because you are undertaking a professional and academic programme of study and development, there are specific learning objectives to be achieved. In a typical health-care curriculum, course philosophy, aims, objectives/learning outcomes and content are influenced, if not decided, by a combination of agencies. These include professional bodies, the academic validation process, the course planners themselves, students, government initiatives/demands, prevailing social, political, ethical, legal, economic, health promotion and disease considerations, plus other current philosophical considerations affecting patient care.

Portfolios should be informative and authentic

Good portfolios are informative, meaningful and intelligible to read. They must be meaningful to all stakeholders. Ask yourself who the people with an interest in your portfolio are and what they will be looking for. Will it be intelligible to them?

Key points Top tips

- Portfolios should be informative and authentic

Is the portfolio authentic? Is it based on true self-assessment of the producer's needs? Are claims substantiated? Is evidence sound, clear and authenticated where this is considered necessary? Are the learning activities and reflections based on personal experiential components?

Finally, a good portfolio will acknowledge limitations on the part of you as the writer. It may point out limitations in the portfolio development and compilation process and how such limitations have affected the final product. It may even suggest recommendations for further learning and development, for your own benefit as well as for the reader.

Over to you

You are asked to assess the portfolio of a peer who is undertaking a preregistration health-care diploma or degree programme similar to your own.
- Draw up an assessment and marking plan containing the points you would look for in the portfolio.
- Offer a critical discussion that explains your reasoning and rationale for the marking criteria you have drawn up on your plan.

Key points | Top tips

- It is essential that the arrangement of a portfolio is clear, well-articulated and highly structured.
- A contents page, together with a clear outline of the arrangement of the portfolio and exactly where to find relevant evidence, is absolutely crucial.
- Clearly articulated reasons must be provided to justify anything put into the portfolio.
- It is difficult to specify word limit. As the writer of the portfolio, you usually determine its size. However, if the course or developmental programme to which your portfolio is linked specifies a word limit, be sure to follow this. A very big portfolio does not necessarily signify a good or bad portfolio; quality is what matters.
- A good portfolio identifies personal development needs and how they are addressed. It concentrates on past, present and future development perspectives. It contains clear supporting evidence and uses a critical reflective approach. It shows respect for any imposed specific learning outcomes and, where appropriate, follows course and other developmental programme guidelines and marking criteria.
- Assessments of portfolios in learning and development must recognise the individual nature of a person's portfolio. Assessment must show respect for individuality, student choice, autonomy and self-determination.

Assessing actual and potential credit values of a portfolio

Professional bodies

A number of agencies may well have an interest in assessing the actual and potential credit value of the portfolio of a health-care student or qualified health-care professional. A health-care student such as a nurse needs to be aware that their professional body (the NMC) actually makes it a requirement that they develop a professional portfolio as a means of advancing their professional development and practice. The requirement applies both in the preregistration education and training phase and at qualified practitioner level following registration.

The development of portfolios by nurses and physiotherapists (for example) is therefore not a passing fad! Neither is it done just for the purpose of passing a diploma or degree course and gaining professional registration. The expectation that these groups will continue to develop their portfolio beyond registration is enshrined in policies made by their professional bodies. It is a necessary requirement throughout the span of their professional careers. For qualified nurses in particular, continued development and professional portfolio building are tied into criteria-linked periodic re-licensing/re-registration. What does this really mean?

Put simply, when nurses first pass their preregistration course, whether at diploma or degree level, they gain eligibility for professional body registration. To register they pay a fee, currently to the NMC. At the time of writing, initial registration lasts 3 years, after which a further fee has to be paid to maintain suitability and credibility to practise. However suitability and credibility to practise are not based solely on the ability to pay the re-licensing fee. Every registered nurse and physiotherapist must be able to demonstrate evidence of continued professional development in order to maintain their registration and practise status. Continued portfolio development is one of the main ways of demonstrating this.

Postregistration education and practice

As indicated above, under the NMC's Postregistration education and practice (PREP) policy, all nurses are expected to demonstrate evidence of continued professional development. Continued portfolio development will facilitate this and is a sound way to show that your learning has not become stale, underdeveloped or out of touch. The NMC considers it an obligation, and indeed a legal responsibility, to ensure that nurses on the professional register remain suitable to continue to practise. This body can at any time demand to see a nurse's professional portfolio. This is not to say that your portfolio at the postqualifying level will be the only means by which you can demonstrate evidence of continuing development, but it will be a very credible document to use to support your claims of continued educational and practice development before and after registration. Do not be found wanting by not updating yourself and your portfolio!

Another occasion when an assessment and evaluation of your portfolio may take place is if, as a health-care professional, you apply to get on to an advanced academic and professional development programme. Under the credit accumulation and transfer (CAT) scheme, you may wish to apply for exemption from certain modules or elements of the programme you have applied for. Your portfolio could be an excellent authoritative source of evidence to the effect that you already possess the knowledge, skills and competencies you seek to be credited with. In this way you could find yourself doing the new programme in a shortened period of time. You may also save yourself some money on course fees and avoid the boredom arising from repeating things that you have done before.

A related point worth mentioning here concerns the notions of accreditation of prior learning (APL) and accreditation of prior experiential learning (APEL). Under APL, you may seek and gain recognition for previous learning. Under APEL you may also be able to seek accreditation for prior experiential learning. Your portfolio may again come in useful at this point, being used to assess your credibility for claim to APL and APEL.

It is so important to continue to develop your portfolio beyond professional registration. If you have (in your portfolio) programme and module guides, student handbooks, other written and authenticated summary breakdowns of courses and professional development programmes you have previously followed, you have yet more assessable elements that can help you make the case for recognition of your previous learning and experience. Reading this, can you honestly say, yes, I have kept intact all the module guides that were given to me on my diploma or degree course? Your portfolio has much credit value, not only at preregistration but also at postregistration level.

Academic credits and levels

Educational credits and levels are summarised in Table 4.2. When you undertake an undergraduate degree programme of study you work through three academic levels before you quality for your degree. Let us take as a reference point a 3-year degree programme. Normally, year 1 is achieved at academic level 1 or certificate level,

Table 4.2 Portfolio assessment by programme year, academic level and credit value

Year	Academic level	Academic credits
Year 1	Portfolio assessed at level 1 (Certificate)	Determined by programme or module specification
Year 2	Portfolio assessed at level 2 (Diploma)	Determined by programme or module specification
Year 3	Portfolio assessed at level 2 or 3 (Diploma or Degree)	Determined by programme or module specification

year 2 at academic level 2 or diploma level, and year 3 at academic level 3 or degree level.

If you have had portfolio work summatively assessed in years 1, 2 and 3, then the assessment will usually have taken place through the three academic levels. It is useful to note here, however, that certain 'undergraduate' nursing programmes, for example, confer Master's ('M' level) degrees on successful candidates. Theoretically, then, if a health-care student's portfolio, or elements of it, have been assessed at 'M' level, in reality s/he has some 'M' level credits linked to that portfolio.

There is also the concept of academic credits for modules and whole programmes. You may recall seeing '10 credits', '20 credits' or '30 credits' written on module guides. The number of credits given for a module depends on a number of factors – e.g. the amount of work done, the number of teaching hours, teacher-student contact hours and hours spent in self-directed study. If your portfolio has been the only summative assessment requirement to pass a given module, then the portfolio is credited with the total number of academic credits allocated to that module.

Key points / **Top tips**

- Find out from your course planners and educators just how many academic credits your portfolio attracted for a particular module.
- It may well be that your portfolio forms only part of your module assessment. If this is the case, your course director or the examinations officer should normally be able to tell you what percentage of the total modular credits your portfolio has attracted.

The quality, level and difficulty index of learning outcomes influence academic levels of attainment. But what does this mean? If your learning outcomes are pitched at the higher levels of knowledge attainment (e.g. at analysis, synthesis, problem solving and evaluation), you are more likely to secure level 3 credits than if they are pitched at the lower levels of knowledge (e.g. recall of knowledge, memorising facts, basic descriptions and uncritical application of facts). When submitting your portfolio for assessment at degree level and beyond, you must remember to demonstrate evidence of learning, professional and academic growth, with reference to at least some of the higher-level action verbs – analyse, evaluate, etc. In other words, critically evaluate and analyse your growth and development and produce critical reflective supportive evidence.

Critical level 3 reflections recorded in your portfolio must show evidence that you have been able to analyse, critically, the issues involved, taking account of legal, ethical/moral and political considerations and their influence on clinical decision making. In Chapter 2 of this book you came across the concept of Goodman's levels of reflection. Level 3 calls for health-care professionals to be able to examine how issues of 'justice', autonomy and freedom influence critical discussions about professional goals and practice. Level 3 also requires the health-care clinician to make links between everyday practice realities and the wider socioeconomic realities and constraints operating at the time.

Another agency that may well feel it has a right and an obligation to examine your portfolio or profile is your employer. Employers of nurses and other health-care professionals are duty-bound to ensure that people practising in their employ are suitably qualified and currently registered with their professional registration body. This means that your NHS manager, for example, could call upon you at any time to produce evidence showing that you are still a registered practitioner and that you have indeed continued to update yourself for practice purposes. Once again, it can be seen that the assessment of your portfolio and, through the portfolio, the evaluation of your own professional development is of crucial importance.

Potential employers may also wish to see your portfolio as a means of helping them decide on your suitability for employment. Indeed, you may be so proud of your portfolio that you may decide to offer it for inspection. You may already be familiar with the concept of life-long learning and the obligation put on health-care professionals to demonstrate evidence of this. What better way for you to demonstrate this than through your up-to-date portfolio?

Hopefully you can now see the value to you and your patients of a dynamic and up-to-date portfolio. You have so many agencies with an interest in your portfolio, not to mention its positive contribution to your critical review of your own practice and professional development needs, that you should ensure that it is always ready to stand up to critical scrutiny. It is indeed a learning and professional development tool in your pre- and postregistration education and practice. It has the potential to help you come through all assessment and evaluation of your learning, professional growth and practice.

Reflective activity

Reflect critically on the importance of a health-care student developing and maintaining a portfolio pre- and postregistration.

Over to you

You have been asked to use your portfolio to undertake a short but critical reflection on an experience you have had in education or clinical practice.

- Carry out the reflection and write it down in your portfolio.
- Ask one of your peers or your personal tutor to provide you with a written, critical opinion on your written reflection. Insert this written critique in your portfolio, together with your own reflection on it.

Key points Top tips

- Although a variety of interested parties, bodies and agencies may exercise claim to your professional portfolio and/or profile, it is still a personal private document.
- The fact that a portfolio is so versatile shows its importance.
- A portfolio may be the ideal vehicle for you to use to seek credit for prior learning and prior experiential learning and development within national credit accumulation and transfer schemes.
- A portfolio may be assessed in relation to both academic credit values and academic levels.
- Portfolios create an opportunity to engage in life-long learning.
- As a health-care professional, a portfolio may be at the heart of your ability to grow and develop professionally and personally. It may even influence your ability to impress your employer and potential employers.

> ## ⌐⌐⌐⌐⌐⌐*Rapid recap*
>
> Check your progress so far by working through each of the following questions.
>
> 1. Explain the difference between a formative and summative assessment.
> 2. List four sets of modifying factors that assessors should take into consideration when assessing a student's portfolio.
> 3. What are the notions of accreditation of prior learning (APL) and accreditation of prior experiential learning (APEL)?
>
> If you have difficulty with more than one of the questions, read through the section again to refresh your understanding before moving on.

References

Biggs, J. (1979) Individual difference in study processes and the quality of learning outcomes. *Higher Education*, **8**, 381–394.

Biggs, J. (1999) *Teaching for Quality Learning at University*. SRHE/Open University Press, Buckingham.

Department for Education and Employment (1991) *National Records of Achievement*. DfEE, London.

Department for Education and Skills (2002) *Progress File*. DfES, London.

Flood, J. and Lapp, D. (1989) Reporting reading progress: a comparison portfolio for parents. *Reading Teacher*, **42**, 508–514.

Jongsma, K. S. (1989) Portfolio assessment. *Reading Teacher*, **43**, 264–265.

Moya, S. S. and O'Malley, J. M. (1994) A portfolio assessment model for ESL. *Journal of Educational Issues of Language Minority Students*, **13**, 13–36.

Tiwari, A. and Tang, C. (2003) Does portfolio assessment encourage students to adopt different assessment preparation strategies? Online at http://www.ugc.edu.hk/tlqpr01/site/abstracts/068_tiwari1.htm (accessed February 2003)

Valencia, S. W. (1990a) A portfolio approach to classroom reading assessment: the whys, whats, and hows. *Reading Teacher*, **43**, 338–340.

Valencia, S. W. (1990b). Alternative assessment: separating the wheat from the chaff. *Reading Teacher*, **43**, 60–61.

5

Continuing professional development

Learning outcomes

By the end of this chapter you should be able to:

- Provide a definition for continuing professional development, personal development plans and life-long learning.
- Acknowledge the influence of government policy on continuing professional development.
- Identify the purpose of a professional portfolio in supporting continuing professional development.

This chapter introduces the concepts of practice development, clinical governance, life-long learning, personal development plans and clinical supervision. Once you have started training as a health-care professional you have started a life-long journey of self-development and discovery. Practice development, clinical governance, life-long learning, personal development plans and clinical supervision are all integral components of continuing professional development and you need to understand the driving force behind the campaign for continuing professional development.

You may feel a bit overwhelmed by all the various terminology surrounding government legislation, such as clinical governance, life-long learning, clinical supervision, etc. They are all terms generated by the government, which the professional bodies have then adopted, to ultimately improve the quality of care for clients and enhance the expertise of health-care professionals through effective learning. It is important that you understand or are aware of the politics and subsequent policies that inform your professional practice. Health-care professionals have been criticised in the past for not being particularly politically aware and this needs to change, and has changed since the recognition of many health-care roles as professions.

Practice development

The government requires practitioners who are fit for practice to fulfil their vision of a modern, dependable NHS. As a response to this requirement, many Trusts have formed practice development units. These units are staffed to provide support for practitioners within the Trust, whether they are students, are newly qualified or have been in the Trust for a number of years. The aim of the majority of practice development teams is to enhance client care by focusing on the development of the practitioners responsible for that care.

There has been recent national and local recognition of areas of clinical care in the NHS that could be improved. One of the areas of improvement that clients are most concerned about is basic care, including helping them wash, walk, eat and drink, moving and lifting them, helping them to the toilet, making sure they are comfortable and giving them pain relief. Ward-based staff, including nurses, physiotherapists, occupational therapists, dietitians and speech therapists, perform many of these tasks.

At Addenbrooke's NHS Trust, the specific purpose of practice development is defined as ensuring that all care is:

- Centred on the client (not on the needs of the staff)
- Based on evidence (i.e. based on published data, good practice guidelines and feedback from patients)
- Appropriate for the needs of each patient
- Effective (i.e. 'it works').

At Addenbrooke's, practice development is led by members of the Practice Development Group and is carried out by practice development facilitators; this is common to the majority of Trusts in the country.

You may ask, 'How does this influence my portfolio development?' When you qualify and start working for a Trust you will meet members of the practice development team, who are there to support and advise you. This links to your portfolio, as you can discuss its development with them in terms of increasing knowledge, skills and competence, or career progression.

Clinical governance

In 1998, the government produced a White Paper to determine quality at the heart of health care to ensure that all clients in the NHS received high-quality care. The government then started a 10-year modernisation programme to ensure fair access to prompt high quality care wherever a client is treated. The government has developed partnerships with the clinical professions to establish quality and high standards of care. The intention is to ensure clear, national standards for services, supported by consistent, evidence-based guidance to raise quality standards.

The consultation document *A First Class Service: Quality in the new NHS* set out a framework for quality improvement and fair access in the NHS, the main components of which were:

- Clear national standards for services and treatments, through National Service Frameworks and a new National Institute for Clinical Excellence

- Local delivery of high quality health care, through clinical governance underpinned by modernised, professional self-regulation and extended life-long learning
- Effective monitoring of progress through a new Commission for Health Improvement, a framework for assessing performance in the NHS and a new national survey of patient and user experience.

The term 'clinical governance' has been used in reference to improving quality and is the process by which each part of the NHS quality-assures its clinical decisions. Clinical governance is defined by the Department of Health (1998) as a system through which NHS organisations are accountable for continuously improving the quality of their services and safeguarding high standards of care, by creating an environment in which clinical excellence will flourish. Clinical governance is a framework for all members of the health-care team through which practitioners are accountable for improving the quality of their clinical care and ensuring high standards of practice.

At some stage in your career you will hear references made to quality assurance activities such as clinical audit, clinical supervision, risk assessments, evidence-based practice, research, and complaints and critical incident reporting. Clinical governance unites these measures to ensure that quality is at the heart of client-centred practice.

Clinical governance is central to the agenda laid out in *A First Class Service* (Department of Health 1998). It provides a framework within which local organisations can work to improve and assure the quality of clinical services for clients. The government aim to ensure national quality standards are applied consistently within a new system of clinical governance; through extended life-long learning to ensure that NHS staff are equipped to deliver change and are given the opportunity to maintain and develop their skills and expertise. Clinical governance is the driving force for quality through establishing clear lines of accountability for clinical quality systems and effective processes for identifying and managing risk and addressing poor performance. Above all, though, clinical governance is about changing the culture of the NHS to promote a culture where openness and participation are encouraged, where education and research are properly valued, where people learn from failures and blame is the exception rather than the rule, and where good practice and new approaches are freely shared and willingly received (Department of Health 1998).

You can see now why clinical governance has been included within this chapter, as the government considers continuing professional development and life-long learning to be an integral component of its clinical governance agenda. The Department of Health (1998) defines continuing professional development as a process of life-long learning for all individuals and teams that meets the needs of clients and delivers the health outcomes and health priorities of the NHS and that enables professionals to expand and fulfil their potential. Every single health-care professional has a duty to uphold the principles of clinical governance.

Life-long learning

Another government target is to improve and enhance multidisciplinary working with an aim to enhance holistic client care. Health-care professionals should be working together and sharing ideas, reflections and theories to improve client care, offer best practice and develop their own needs. Life-long learning is a philosophy that is considered essential not only to fulfil the requirements from all the health-care professional bodies but also to develop a flexible and enquiring approach to delivering the best client care.

In November 2001 the Department of Health produced a White Paper called *Working Together – Learning Together: A framework for life-long learning for the NHS*. This paper sets out a framework to recognise, value and realise life-long learning as an essential element of successful individual, team and organisational performance. Life-long learning is primarily about growth and opportunity, about making sure that staff are supported to acquire new skills and realise their potential to help change things for the better. Life-long learning aims to provide health-care professionals with the opportunity to continuously update their skills and knowledge to offer the most modern, effective and high quality care to patients. For example, life-long learning will allow health-care professionals to identify training needs across professions to aid clinical team-working (Department of Health 1998).

The aim of the framework is to ensure that clients and their families benefit from a better qualified and motivated workforce by providing direction for those with responsibility for ensuring that life-long learning develops by clarifying for staff what they can expect from their employer to maximise potential, provide the basis for further local guidance and support to inform staff and modernise education and training. Life-long learning covers all aspects of learning and development for health-care staff, from basic induction to pre- and postregistration education, continuing personal and professional development, management and leadership development.

A number of influences have driven the development of this framework as the diversity of people's lifestyles and cultures and their expectations about work and learning are constantly changing. Life-long learning is not just concerned with learning related to work, it goes one step further than work-based learning. A number of influences have driven the government to formalise life-long learning – changes to the wider world of work, the diversity of people's lifestyles and cultures and their changing expectations about work and learning have to be recognised. The rapidly changing nature of health care reflects a need for career-wide continuing professional development and the capacity not only to adapt to change but also to identify the need for change and to initiate change. The portfolio must therefore include the capacity to promote best practice and to address life-long learning skills.

Life-long learning can be divided into three categories: theoretical, personal and practice-related. Demonstration of the theoretical category occurs within the portfolio, for example, in the presentation of reading, writing and information technology skills. Personal development can be demonstrated within your professional role or outside your professional role as any of the following: arts and crafts, fine arts and music, health and physical activities and travel. Of these, travel, health and physical activities and music are the most common. Travel provides an interesting dimension, with the opportunity it gives for the consideration of different cultures and customs. Life-long learning in the practice arena is the most important category for consideration.

Here is a reflection that depicts a teacher's view on practice and personal life-long learning:

> I think I teach students because I recognise that I still have a long way to go, and if I have a long way to go yet, so do they! I encourage them to continue to mature and grow. I don't know where or why I thought about it, but I've always had the concept that you never arrive at a given point when you say, now I know everything I need to know. Learning and development goes on until death, unless you just give up and do nothing, you know. I think it's possible to keep on developing throughout your life.

Life-long learning participants need to be active learners who engage in a wide variety of self-directed learning opportunities through informal avenues, independent learning projects and other differing resources. The portfolio supports this diversity of learning by

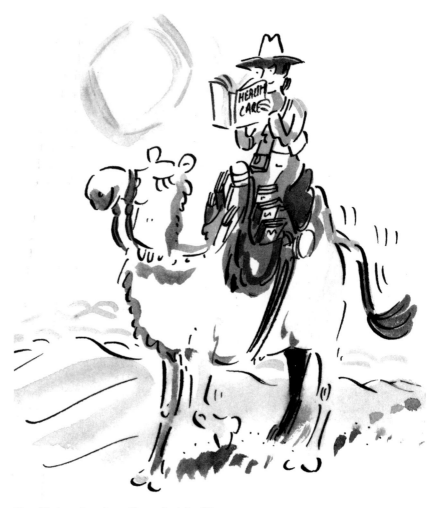

Your life-long learning will manifest itself in many ways

providing a flexible medium in which to consider and demonstrate your learning. Through being an active learner you come to understand that you are responsible for your own learning.

Reflective activity

Consider this reflection and see how you feel about it. Can you relate to what the person is thinking and saying?

'You have to have a little bit of intellectual curiosity that keeps stimulating yourself. I don't think it's automatic. You have to keep on working at it. You have to deliberately decide that you want to keep on. And as you do, one thing leads to another, keeps stimulating. Learning stimulates learning. It keeps you alive. Learning stimulates learning.'

The government, the NHS and health-care professional bodies are all working towards an organisational culture where life-long learning and continuing professional development are seen as key issues for developing a workforce that is fit for practice. The standard statements state that health-care practitioners will engage in self-development to improve knowledge and skills in order to remain competent and practice within a framework that will include a suitable learning environment and appraisal system (Department of Health, 2001). This means that health-care professionals must demonstrate improving their knowledge and developing skills through a process of self-evaluation and reflection on practice, providing written evidence that an assessment of the learning acquired has taken place, identifying and recording engagement in continuing professional development and life-long learning activity, written evidence of personal development plans, maintenance of a professional portfolio and inclusion of an individual performance review. Basically, all the statements listed are part of maintaining a professional portfolio, as they make up the core components of a portfolio.

Key points | **Top tips**

- By keeping an up to date portfolio you will be working towards the government, NHS and professional body agenda of life-long learning.

Personal development plans

A personal development plan can either stand alone as a self-appraisal with goals set and actions planned or it can be part of a more formal appraisal. Developing a personal development plan is always a good idea as it helps to structure and organise your continuing professional development and life-long learning. It should begin with your previous personal development plan but, if you do not have one, a review of your experience to date is a good place to start. You can do this formally, as in an appraisal setting, or by yourself. Begin by considering the following points:

- Assess your current standards of practice – if you are a student you can use your most recent assessment of practice document
- Review past experience and learning – for your first personal development plan this can be the last 3 years (including school if you are a student; any work experience is good); for a follow-up personal development plan this should be the last year

- Evaluate past experience and learning – think about what you have done to keep your clinical practice updated, to expand your clinical skills, to improve your standard of care and to keep yourself motivated

- Appraise your performance and the standards of your knowledge and practice – be objective: there is no point in fooling yourself

- Work through specific areas of interest or learning need

- Having identified your learning needs, begin the process of setting goals, devising action plans to meet them and evaluating the outcomes

- Decide how best to achieve the action plan, including time and resources considerations.

Over to you

Redman (1994) supplies an exercise within his book for individual portfolio development. I have adapted this slightly, as it provides a good basis for a personal development plan. Work through the stages and develop your own plan:

- **Step 1: Previous experience**. Describe your experience either through a reflective account, thoughtful consideration or to an appraiser. Summarise and record the experience.

- **Step 2: Learning from experience**. Consider the learning you have gained from your previous experience either through a reflective account, thoughtful consideration or to an appraiser. Summarise and record the learning.

- **Step 3: Demonstrate competence**. Put together evidence to show how you use the learning that has been recorded. Evidence can be direct examples of your work, through discussion with your appraiser or with others or through written work (direct observation, question and answer or other evidence).

- **Step 4. Learning needs**. List three clinical skills within your current role for which you have not yet demonstrated competence. List three further learning needs that are not clinical skills. If you are an experienced practitioner, you can focus more on the further learning needs

- **Step 5. Developing a learning programme**. Consider which of the continuing learning needs are priorities in terms of importance to current role, importance for your future role and areas of special interest. You then need to prioritise your learning and consider what resources you will need to achieve the learning. Do not be unrealistic in terms of what you can achieve – three competencies or learning needs is enough.

The benefits of a personal development plan are many. Here are some of them:

- Provides practitioners and students with a structured learning opportunity to assist in the development of individual maximum potential.
- Supports transition and development in relation to current practice.
- Assists in developing competency-based skills that are needed and are relevant to practice.
- Advocates effective practice and accountable practitioners by facilitating the development of knowledge, experience and clinical skills.
- Facilitates and supports a negotiated learning experience that focuses on reflection, clinical skills and life-long learning.
- Encourages portfolio development and the use of a portfolio in developing a personal development plan.

Successful personal development planning maximises the potential of every practitioner. Identification of an individual's competence, practice, leadership and clinical potential can be formalised by bringing and creating a personal development plan within an individual performance review. The individual performance review should be carried out in accordance with the local agreement and can be supported by the content of the portfolio and personal development plan.

Clinical supervision

Clinical supervision is a practice-focused professional relationship that enables you to reflect on your practice with the support of a skilled supervisor. Through reflection you can further develop your skills, knowledge and enhance your understanding of your own practice (Nursing and Midwifery Council, 2001). The NHS Management Executive (1993) define clinical supervision as a formal process of professional support and learning that enables individual practitioners to develop knowledge and competence, assume responsibility for their own practice and enhance consumer protection and the safety of care in complex situations. It is central to the process of learning and to the expansion of the scope of practice and should be seen as a means of encouraging self-assessment and analytic and reflective skills.

Clinical supervision assists practitioners to develop skills, knowledge and professional values throughout their careers. This enables them to develop a deeper understanding of what it is to be an accountable practitioner and to link to the reality of practice more easily than has previously been possible (UKCC, 1996).

The following key points for clinical supervision come from the Nursing and Midwifery Council but are applicable to all health-care professionals.

1. Clinical supervision supports practice, enabling practitioners to maintain and promote standards of care.

2. Clinical supervision is a practice-focused professional relationship involving a practitioner reflecting on practice with a skilled supervisor.

3. Practitioners and managers according to local circumstances should develop the process of clinical supervision. Ground rules should be agreed so that practitioners and supervisors approach clinical supervision openly, confidently and are aware of what is involved.

4. Every practitioner should have access to clinical supervision. Each supervisor should supervise a realistic number of practitioners.

5. Preparation for supervisors can be effected using 'in-house' or external education programmes. The principles and relevance of clinical supervision should be included in pre- and postregistration education programmes.

6. Evaluation of clinical supervision is needed to assess how it influences care, practice standards and the service.

7. Evaluation systems should be determined locally.

Clinical supervision is not supposed to be carried out within a hierarchy. It is not a managerial concern or a managerial responsibility. The benefits of clinical supervision are considered to be:

- Maintenance and promotion of standards of care
- Reflection on practice
- Life-long learning
- Risk management
- Improved staff morale
- Improved recruitment and retention.

The potential influence on the quality of client care and continuing professional development is considered to be sufficient to merit investment in clinical supervision.

Clinical supervision can help you to develop your skills and knowledge throughout your career. It is an integral part of your life-long learning. It should be available to you throughout your career, enabling you to constantly evaluate and improve your contribution to client care. Clinical supervision aims to bring practitioners and skilled supervisors together to reflect on practice, to identify solutions to problems, to increase understanding of professional issues and, most importantly, to improve standards of care.

One of the main reasons for introducing clinical supervision is to help the process of continuing professional development, life-long learning, effective change management and improved practice. Continuing professional development and clinical supervision are an important part of clinical governance.

Among other health-care professions, dietetics has come to the fore as an autonomous profession, changing fundamental preregistration and postregistration training to reflect the changing roles and responsibilities expected of the dietitian in modern practice (British Dietetic Association, 1991). Most health-care professions are implementing clinical supervision. It is not intended to replace management, mentors or personal development plans. It is a process to facilitate support, encourage professional growth and improve client care.

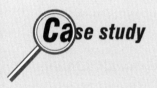

Case study

Unreasonable workload

This is a practice problem that will no doubt arise at some point in your career – **you feel you are being asked to take on an unreasonable workload**. Listed below are the different support mechanisms that should be available to help you tackle the problem.

Manager	You would expect your manager to attempt to alleviate the problem or to explain why such a workload has been placed upon you.
Mentor	You would expect your mentor, if you have one, to listen to you and perhaps provide you with suggestions as to how you can deal with the situation. S/he might suggest that it needs discussion with your manager.
Personal development plan	You could identify and reflect upon your increased workload as an issue in your personal development plan and develop strategies for dealing with the issue. This may involve better time management skills or identification of areas of further development that will assist you in dealing with an increased workload – i.e. increasing confidence in being able to ask for help from colleagues or enhancing your skills to facilitate ease of workload.

Case study continued

Clinical supervision

You would discuss the issues with your supervisor and explore your feelings and attitudes towards the increased workload. You might consider some possible solutions together but the main focus would be discussing you, how you feel and how you are coping. You would not expect your clinical supervisor to do anything practically about the situation.

Whichever route of support you choose, and you may choose more than one, the process of asking for help and the outcome of that help should be reflected upon and submitted as evidence in your portfolio.

Continuing professional development

Continuing professional development is the process by which professionals update, maintain and enhance their knowledge and expertise in order to ensure their competence to practice. Continuing professional development is a systematic and ongoing process.

British Dietetic Association, 1998

The health-care professions comprise an extensive and diverse range of personnel, including nurses, physiotherapists, dietitians, radiographers, podiatrists, occupational therapists, drama therapists, music therapists, art therapists and prosthetic therapists, to name but a few. The level of education, type of work carried out and the amount of responsibility varies a great deal within and across the professions. In the UK, health-care professionals generally work in the primary care or acute care trusts, or within the private sector, and work alongside each other, so there has to be a certain amount of inter- and multidisciplinary working.

Changes in the way in which health-care professionals are perceived, along with changes in health-care organisation, have created an environment in which individual health-care professionals must take control of their future professional development and careers. Educators, employers and professional organisations also have a key role to play in nurturing the professional development of health-care professionals.

Continuing professional development activity can take many forms, but fostering a personal culture in which development is inherent in everyday working practices is especially valuable. Reflection and portfolio development needs to be an intrinsic part of your practice to help you to expand your own knowledge and understanding of it. At the end of the day, these activities will probably save you time, because the learning achieved and the changes you make to your practice are immediate.

Factors that can restrict continuing professional development include lack of time, resources, support and recognition. However, the government, professional bodies and health-care organisations now take the continuing professional development of health-care professionals very seriously, driven by the need for an accountable, competent and flexible workforce.

Health-care professionals need to incorporate professional development into their role to remain competent, relevant and clinically effective. They must take ownership and be accountable for their own self-development, through a process of self-evaluation and reflection on practice, and for identifying their own continuous professional development requirements. However, many practitioners and students feel uncomfortable with the emphasis on portfolio development and may not understand its relevance in today's practice or where to start to develop the necessary skills.

In the modern NHS, health-care professionals work in a climate of endless change, the expectation being that they will continually rise to new challenges. Continuing professional development is essential in today's work environment. Redman (1994) states that there is increasing recognition for the key attributes needed by people in a constantly changing work environment; these are:

- Communication skills
- Flexibility
- Self-motivation
- Willingness and ability to develop new skills.

If you consider the above fundamental characteristics you can begin to see what is needed within a portfolio to assist and demonstrate development of these key attributes. Portfolios are vital not only for proving that you are continually developing but also for shaping and guiding how you develop. As previously discussed, Redman (1994) describes five stages in portfolio and professional development:

1. Describing experience: the story
2. Identifying learning from experience: the discovery
3. The demonstration of practice: the proof
4. Establishing learning needs: ownership
5. Identifying and taking up learning opportunities: growth and review.

Regardless of your experience, whether you are a young or a mature student or practitioner, by beginning with your experience you can then tell the story.

Over to you

With a colleague, talk about a recent or old experience, for example your first day at university or work experience. Move through Redman's (1994) stages and write down the experience and what you think about it. By going through this process you may identify areas that need development.

Models of continuing professional development

In essence, the portfolio is a vehicle for structuring continuous professional development (British Dietetic Association, 1999). This section gives you three models of continuing professional development that offer strategies to encourage responsibility for engaging in the ongoing process of portfolio development, continuing professional development and life-long learning.

Portfolio development and continuing professional development are obviously interlinked, as the portfolio is usually the medium in which you record your continuing professional development; therefore it needs to be a dynamic process. Continuing professional development begins the moment you start your professional training and a brief look at Benner's model of skills acquisition may be useful to illustrate the need to start thinking about it immediately. Benner (1984) identifies five levels of reflection in her model:

- Stage 1: Novice
- Stage 2: Advanced beginner
- Stage 3: Competent
- Stage 4: Proficient
- Stage 5: Expert.

Benner's model has been adapted for many different purposes within the health-care professions (e.g. it was used as a continuous assessment of practice document for nursing students), as it embraces the concept of moving from novice to expert as your experience increases. The stages are not steps that you continually climb up – an experienced practitioner moving into a new clinical area with no prior experience may be practising at the 'novice' level. Similarly, a student who has just completed a practice placement in an acute specialty may be considered 'competent' but moving to the next placement within a different specialty will bring the student back to the 'novice' level. The five stages are useful for assessing what level you are at so you know where to begin in relation to your continuing professional development, personal development plan and subsequent portfolio development.

Benner's model exhibits similarities to the educational model of Blake and Blanchard (Pemberton, 1999), which identifies four levels of learning:

- **Level 1: Unconsciously incompetent**. The practitioner 'doesn't know what they don't know' and is therefore unaware. This is the 'I teach, you learn' stage, where the clinical mentor/supervisor is the 'teacher' (Novice)
- **Level 2: Consciously incompetent**. The practitioner is aware but hasn't developed the skills to practise safely. This is the 'you learn and I help' stage, where the mentor/supervisor is the 'coach' (Advanced beginner)
- **Level 3: Consciously competent**. The practitioner is aware and able to function effectively but the skills are not yet automatic. This is the 'let's learn' stage, where the mentor/supervisor facilitates learning (Competent/proficient)
- **Level 4: Unconsciously competent**. Skills are so deeply ingrained as to be automatic/intuitive, demonstrating reflection-in-action. This is the 'I need to know' stage, where the mentor/supervisor becomes a consultant, providing access to information (Expert).

Figure 5.1 shows the model for continuing professional development produced by the Department of Health (1999):

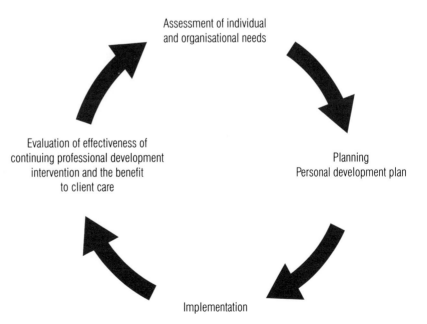

Figure 5.1 *Model of continuing professional development (Department of Health, 1999)*

Benner's skills acquisition model, the educational model of Blake and Blanchard and the Department of Health model of professional development provide a useful theoretical base for continuing professional development. The majority of health-care practitioner employers will help as much as possible by providing the necessary support and education but the responsibility for continuing professional development rests with the individual, who needs to lead the process.

To demonstrate how continuing professional development and personal development plans interact with each other, the following points need to be considered for the process of continuing professional development:

- Identifying developmental needs
- Planning how these needs are best met
- Implementing action plans
- Applying learning/theory to practice
- Evaluating the benefits of that application of learning
- Identifying and planning further needs.

The ultimate aims of professional development and portfolio development are the same – to improve the quality of patient care by the ongoing development of competent practitioners. It is therefore feasible to use the process of professional development as a means of fulfilling the requirements for portfolio development, and *vice versa*.

RRRRR**Rapid recap**

Check your progress so far by working through each of the following questions.

1. How is the specific purpose of practice development defined at Addenbrooke's NHS Trust?
2. Name the three categories of life-long learning.
3. What is clinical supervision?
4. Why do health-care professionals need to incorporate professional development into their role?

If you have difficulty with more than one of the questions, read through the section again to refresh your understanding before moving on.

References

Benner, P. (1984) *From Novice to Expert: Excellence and power in clinical nursing practice*. Addison-Wesley, Menlo Park, CA.

British Dietetic Association (1991) *Towards the 21st Century – A consultation document*. BDA, Birmingham.

British Dietetic Association (1998) *Continuing Professional Development for Dieticians – Policy paper*. BDA, Birmingham.

British Dietetic Association (1999) *A Professional Portfolio for Dietitians*. BDA, Birmingham.

Department of Health (1998) *A First Class Service: Quality in the new NHS*. DOH, London.

Department of Health (1999) *Continuing Professional Development: Quality in the new NHS*. DOH, London.

Department of Health (2001) *Working Together – Learning Together: A framework for lifelong learning for the NHS*. DOH, London.

NHS Management Executive (1993) *A Vision for the Future: The nursing, midwifery and health visiting contribution to health and health care*. DOH, London.

Nursing and Midwifery Council (2001) *Clinical Supervision*. NMC, London

Pemberton, I. (1999) The 4 levels of learning. *Training Solutions*, **6**, 28–31.

Redman, W. (1994) *Portfolios for Development*. Kogen Page. London.

UK Central Council (1994) *The Future of Professional Practice: The Council's standards for education and practice following registration*. UKCC, London.

UK Central Council (1996) *Position Statement on Clinical Supervision for Nursing and Health Visiting*. UKCC, London.

6

Continuing with your professional portfolio

Learning outcomes

By the end of this chapter you should be able to:

- Understand the need for continuing with your portfolio
- Understand the importance of your portfolio in terms of your continuing professional development
- Consider your skills inventory in relation to your job and understand how this can inform your portfolio.

Particularly with an assessed portfolio, there is a tendency, once it has served the purpose for which it was intended, for it to be left to gather dust on a shelf. I hope one of the points you have taken from this book so far is that reflection and portfolio development are an essential part of your practice and support how you learn and promote best practice. There may be times when you feel less enthused about your development and your portfolio, and this is understandable. However, try not to leave it for too long. Once you are in the habit of making regular entries it is easier to keep this pattern going.

Redfern (1998) says that a well-kept portfolio provides us with a detailed map of our professional lives and that in the busyness of everyday life we tend to forget what we have achieved, concentrating on what we haven't done well or what's gone wrong. I believe this to be a very important observation. I occasionally look back at my own portfolio from my Masters degree and find it incredible that I learnt all that I did during that time. It is also beneficial by showing me how I have moved on and how I have used the knowledge, skills and competence gained then to enhance my practice and my career.

Once your portfolio has been assessed or submitted to a professional body, or has supported you through an interview, you may then ask, 'How do I carry on?'

I would suggest that, for all portfolios, regardless of their intended purpose, you aim to provide a triangulation of evidence with each submission. By this I mean that you use experiences from practice, linked to a theoretical component and then backed with evidence-based practice or current literature. Reflections or portfolio entries need to be supported by reference to sources of information, informed by external data to include research literature, evidence-based practice tools, government legislation, requirements of professional bodies and local and national policy. For example, when discussing or reflecting on client care you can do so in the context of the **National Service Frameworks**.

⊶ᴛ *Keywords*

National Service Frameworks

'Care blueprints' that define how services are best provided and to what standard

The government wants to establish national standards for the foremost health problems in the UK – coronary heart disease, cancer and mental health are three of the areas identified.

To reaffirm the importance of supporting your evidence with appropriate facts, another model for supporting your portfolio evidence may be useful. This links to the triangulation of evidence model given in Chapter 2:

- **Learning for practice**; represents *theory and education*, which includes professional development courses/modules and study/theory days
- **Learning while practising**; represents *experience*, which includes personal and professional development through reflection, personal development plans, reflection-in-action and reflection-on-action
- **Learning through practice**; represents *evidence-based practice and literature*, which includes evidence-based practice and practice-based projects/research.

Student portfolios – the transition to professional practice

The transition from student to qualified practitioner is a stressful yet exciting time. There are many opportunities for portfolio development within the first year of qualifying – it is a key stage in your development and should be recorded, as it charts what is likely to be the steepest learning curve in your career.

When you begin a new job there are certain experiences that are inevitable, and these should be documented in your portfolio – you will attend a Trust induction day or equivalent and meet your identified mentor to negotiate your personal development plan or appraisal, identifying individual goals relating to professional development and life-long learning and working alongside your mentor when possible.

Most important are your feelings about being newly qualified. How does it feel to be accountable for your actions? Do you feel supported to take on this new accountability? Do you feel ready? There will inevitably be gaps in your training. The nature of health-care means that learning is continuous and you will never be fully prepared for qualification, but you should feel that, through fostering a deep approach to learning and portfolio development, you have basic and guiding principles on which to act and with which to practise safely.

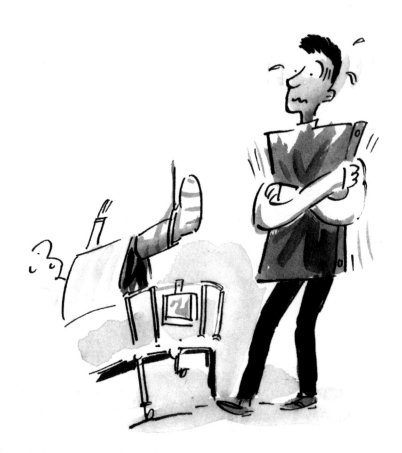

Knowing you have completed your student portfolio may give you more confidence when you finally become qualified

When you qualify you may wonder what to do with your student portfolio. It is an ideal starting point for your postqualification portfolio. Whether it was assessed or not is irrelevant in terms of its usefulness after you qualify. Do not start a brand new portfolio when you qualify, you need to use the key factors about yourself from your student portfolio to inform your personal development plans and subsequent professional career.

Key points | **Top tips**

- Remember that a portfolio is about recording personal and professional growth – this needs to be evident in your postqualification portfolio.
- When you qualify, you do not start at the beginning again, you have skills and knowledge acquired during training and these must be carried over.

You need to gather the information from your student portfolio that is relevant to qualification (e.g. skills inventories, latest practice documents, most recent reflections and any information that is pertinent to qualified practice).

If you feel comfortable with the structure of your student portfolio it makes sense to remain with it. Check that the terminology within a 'ready-made' student portfolio is appropriate for a postqualification portfolio. By this I mean that it does not refer to working towards prequalification competencies. If the section headings are appropriate but the detail within the sections is not, keep the section headings and consider how your job description fits within each section.

Table 6.1 on the next page shows some generic job description headings, which can be considered as a skills inventory. I have linked the skills listed to the sections suggested in Example 1 in Chapter 8 to demonstrate how they can be incorporated.

The purpose of the skills inventory is to provide you with a benchmark of what you should be working towards as a practitioner. It is generic and at a relatively basic level. For a more detailed skills inventory aimed at the level appropriate for your expertise, you should refer to your own job description.

Keeping a skills inventory, a clinical practice record, your personal development plans and a review of your clinical placements once qualified will provide a record of your achievements and targeted areas for development. There are also many relevant points within the skills inventory that can be easily linked to government policy, professional body requirements and evidence-based practice tools.

Chapter 3 discussed reflecting on the context in which the care is given. This incorporates considering the wider social structure but also adds a social caring perspective. Reference to external issues will add depth and weight to any reflective or non-reflective entry – considering the wider picture during your reflections can demonstrate reflective level 3 of Goodman's model. You should attempt to reflect on each portfolio entry on the basis of the context in which the care is being delivered. This includes the external issues surrounding the care, but also the following key points (Walsh, 2000):

- Interpersonal relationships
- External environment, culture
- Involvement – health promotion
- Emotional, psychological and social – relationships, interactions, physical surroundings
- Patient perspective

Table 6.1 Linking a job description to your portfolio

Individualised care	● Be able to assess, plan, implement and evaluate individual programmes of care, taking into account specific needs	Care delivery, Section 2
Case management	● Be able to record care using a problem-solving approach	Care management, Section 3
	● Be able to manage a caseload of clients	Care management, Section 3
Leadership	● Be able to act as a professional role model	Personal and professional development, Section 4
	● Be able to assist in the setting and monitoring of professional standards of care	Professional and ethical practice, Section 1
Teaching/mentoring	● Develop mentorship skills	Personal and professional development, Section 4
	● Teach learners, department assistants, patients and significant others, to obtain the required level of knowledge	Personal and professional development, Section 4
Client advocacy	● Be able to clearly present the client's points of view to others	Professional and ethical practice, Section 1
Professional practice	● Be aware of current research/approaches to patient care, and demonstrate in practice	Care delivery, Section 2
	● Participate in departmental research programmes	Personal and professional development, Section 4
Teamwork	● Be able to work effectively within a team	Care management, Section 3
	● Co-ordinate the activities of the team in the unplanned absence of senior staff	Care management, Section 3
Communication	● Be able to communicate effectively both verbally and in writing within the multidisciplinary team and with clients and their relatives	Care delivery, Section 2
Self-assurance	● Demonstrate the confidence to present own and patient's point of view	Care management, Section 3
Maintain standards	● Maintain the consistency of standard set	Care management, Section 3
	● Be able to take appropriate action if standards are not being met	Care management, Section 3
Initiator	● Be able to contribute new ideas to improve client care	Care delivery, Section 2
	● Demonstrate an ability to successfully adopt and manage change	Care management, Section 3
Self-management	● Be able to prioritise, self-start and self-motivate	Personal and professional development, Section 4
	● Maintain awareness of professional and organisational developments	Personal and professional development, Section 4
	● Recognise personal strengths and weaknesses	Personal and professional development, Section 4

Table 6.1 (continued)		
	● Recognise personal workload limitations and take appropriate action	Personal and professional development, Section 4
Interpersonal	● Be able to interact with clients/visitors and colleagues in a professional and approachable manner	Care delivery, Section 2
Professional conduct	● Be aware of and maintain professional standards of conduct as per professional code	Professional and ethical practice, Section 1
Organisational conduct	● Be aware of and maintain standards of organisational conduct, i.e. uniform policy, reliability, punctuality, health and safety, equal opportunities and other hospital policies	Professional and ethical practice, Section 1 and Care management, Section 3
Budgeting	● Be able to demonstrate budgetary awareness in the planning and implementation of care	Care management, Section 3
Objective setting	● Be able to assist and participate in departmental objective setting ● Demonstrate a willingness to work towards unit and department objectives	Personal and professional development, Section 4 Personal and professional development, Section 4
Problem solving	● Demonstrate the ability to problem-solve in relation to patient care	Care management, Section 3
Training/development	● Be able to recognise the development needs of unqualified and junior personnel and take appropriate action	Personal and professional development, Section 4
Manpower planning	● Demonstrate an understanding of skills mix implications when, for example, planning duty rotas, delegating tasks	Care management, Section 3

- Universal human rights
- Communication – needs critical reflection
- Health promotion, maintenance and restoration
- Advisor, counsellor and collaborator.

These key points can be linked to Goodman's levels of reflection by pinpointing an appropriate level for each objective. The key points might also be guidelines for the content of your portfolio, as they embrace many of the key concepts related to caring in a health-care profession. The evidence they would produce, however, would be inter-related and perhaps difficult to allocate to any particular section. While all portfolios contain duplication of evidence in different sections, these key points are so closely interlinked that it would be difficult to use them as discrete sections.

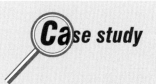

Two levels of reflection

The following are two reflections on a similar incident.

Example 1

A child with eczema was admitted to our ward but the eczema was not the principle reason for admission. There was a lack of appropriate care planning for the management of the eczema. It is important for nurses to be careful not to do everything for the child and that they allow the parents to continue their care. The parent bathed their child in too hot a bath and did not apply the appropriate cream immediately after the bath but this was probably because they were preoccupied with the child's primary complaint. I didn't feel able to say anything as the parents were feeling very vulnerable and I wanted to be supportive and not criticise them. I did feel I didn't think of the child's real needs but it was a balance between the child and the parents and the child did not seem particularly distressed about their eczema and the parents were applying some cream.

Example 2

I was in the situation the other day when a child was admitted to our ward with an asthma attack, when the child had improved I became aware that the child had quite bad eczema although this was not identified on the child's care plan. Peters (2000) states the patient with eczema can present with several features namely, redness and swelling, papules, vesicles, large blisters, exudation and crusting and scaling. The medical staff and the parents seemed largely unaware of treating the child's eczema and this concerned me so after consulting a colleague I decided to contact the paediatric Dermatology Specialist Nurse. Gill (1998) states nurses are playing a greater role in influencing choices of eczema treatment, both in the hospital setting and in the community. The parents did apply emollient cream to the child but they did not use emollients in the bath or a steroid cream as they were concerned about the use of steroids on their child. After the specialist dermatology nurse had assessed the child, he then spent time with the parents informing them of the correct course of treatment and how and when to correctly apply the creams. The parents were concerned about the use of steroid cream but as Gill (1998) states it is often better to use a slightly higher potency steroid to gain control, than to use a weaker steroid for a long period without maximum benefit. The specialist nurse reassured the parents about the use of steroids and it came to light their GP had prescribed steroid cream but they had not used it due to their concern and they had not been given any information regarding how to apply it, its actions or the benefits of using steroids. Peters (2000) states dermatology care is a combination of education about the disease, explaining the role of the topical therapies and demonstrating how they are applied. I felt pleased I had contacted the specialist nurse as he provided valuable support for the parents, he got the medical staff to prescribe a treatment regime and I learnt a lot from spending time with him and feel more confident now when dealing with children with eczema. When I next nurse a child with eczema I will endeavour to ensure the correct care plan is set in place and refer to a specialist colleague if needed.

References

Gill, S. (1998) Use of topical steroids in childhood eczema. *British Journal of Dermatology Nursing*. Winter, 10–11.

Peters, J (2000) Eczema. *Nursing Standard*, **14**(16), 49–55.

Reflective activity

What are the differences between the two examples in terms of level of reflection and the key points discussed above?

The difference between the two reflections should be quite obvious and should demonstrate the different levels of reflection and how they is achieved. If you aim to provide a triangulation of evidence for each reflective entry, with a clear reason as to why you have submitted a particular piece of evidence within your portfolio, your portfolio will address the key issues of providing evidence of reflection and personal and professional development.

Rapid recap

Check your progress so far by working through each of the following questions.
1. What do the following represent?
   a)   Learning for practice
   b)   Learning while practising
   c)   Learning through practice
2. When you qualify, what should you do with your student portfolio?
If you have difficulty with either of the questions, read through the section again to refresh your understanding before moving on.

References

Redfern, L (1998) In: *Continuing Professional Development in Nursing* (ed. F.M. Quinn). Stanley Thornes, Cheltenham.

Walsh, M. (2000) *Nursing Frontiers: Accountability and the boundaries of care*. Butterworth-Heinemann, Oxford.

7

Your curriculum vitae and job application

Learning outcomes

By the end of this chapter you should be able to:

- Write and present a CV.
- Know how best to complete a job application form.
- Understand how to confidently present your CV and job application form to an employer.

The main aim of this chapter is to provide you with the confidence and the practical skills needed to produce a curriculum vitae (CV). It will also provide you with helpful hints on how to complete your job application form and how best to present your application form with your CV to an employer. A CV is a brief summary of your education and experience with the purpose of getting you an interview, so it must attract an employer's attention. The majority of people have an 'interview suit' or dress smartly to present themselves at interview – a CV is the precursor to your interview suit. You need to present the best of yourself every time you make contact with an employer.

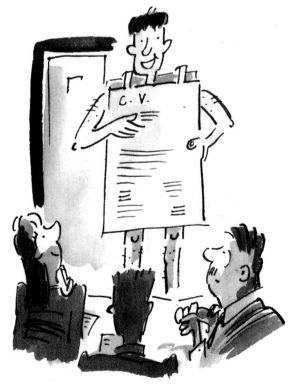

Your CV provides your first point of contact with a potential employer

Top tips

- When a job is likely to attract a lot of interest you have to think like the employer and consider what they want from you.

A CV is a vital part of your portfolio as it provides a condensed version or snapshot of it. It also means you have a ready-made summary of your portfolio to hand should a suitable job be advertised at short notice.

Top tips

There are no set rules on how to present a CV, but it should:
- Attract an employer's interest by being well designed and attractive to look at
- Provide interesting and relevant information
- Sell your key strengths and attributes.

Guiding principles

Writing your CV depends on the purpose for which it is intended. Not all job applications require a CV but it is often valuable to include one as it provides a succinct outline of you and your experience. To determine what to include in your CV consider the following guidelines:

- A CV should be no more than two pages long
- It should be accurate and logical
- It should not be written in the first person – do not use 'I' or 'me'
- Put in a personal statement that highlights the skills and attributes you have and feel are pertinent to the job
- Emphasise from your education and experience what you feel is most relevant
- Exclude information that is immaterial to the job or does not present you in the best light.

Constructing your CV

The headings in your CV should include
- Personal details
- Attributes and skills

- Career history (list the most recent first and work backwards)
- Achievements while in post or in previous posts
- Education and qualifications
- Professional development.

These headings should be altered to suit the job you are applying for. For example, if you have little relevant experience but are well educated, highlight the aspects of your education that you feel the employer will be most interested in. The CD-ROM accompanying this book provides a template for a CV suitable for health-care professionals.

Personal details

This should always be the first heading, although you can put your name and address across the top of the page in one long line (in the 'Header' area provided by Microsoft Word). This type of presentation is useful if you are struggling to save space. Your name should be prominent, either in a larger type or in bold font, and centred e.g.

Sally Smith

1 Sally Smith Street, Sally Smithville, SS1 1SS
Telephone: 0111–111111 E-mail: s.smith@*smithville.co.uk

Other personal details to include:
- Date of birth
- Nationality
- Status.

If the job advertised asks for such things as a car driver or non-smoker, then include these points here.

Attributes and skills

A lot of people who apply for university, or for their first job, feel that they have little experience. Don't be put off if you feel you haven't got a great deal of experience or skills to write about. Everybody has experience in something. Consider what skills you acquired while you were at school or in other employment. For example:
- Studying for exams requires planning and organisation
- Participating in school projects involves teamwork, working to deadlines and often some form of presentation of results
- Have you been a member of a club? Club membership can demonstrate commitment to an organisation and interacting with others

- Do you participate in sport? A team sports player demonstrates an understanding of team dynamics and an ability to communicate with others
- A person who plays non-team sport, e.g. keeping fit, shows commitment and motivation
- Work experience or a part time job can prove ability and development of certain skills – if you have worked in a shop or in a pub/restaurant, for example, you need very good communication and interpersonal skills. This kind of experience is valued in health-care work as it demonstrates an ability to interact with the general public.

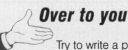

Reflective activity

Think about your key skills and attributes. Compare these skills to those of other people around you. Are there any skills you have that you feel are your particular strengths? Try to list five of them.

Over to you

Try to write a personal statement summarising your key skills – e.g. 'An energetic, self-motivated individual with a keen interest in health care. A resourceful team worker with excellent interpersonal skills, now seeking a more challenging role within a dynamic Trust'.

An employer wants to know how you can use the skills identified in your personal statement to benefit its organisation. These skills are vital pieces of information and you need to ensure that your CV shows them off. If you are writing your CV with a specific job in mind then it should reflect the requirements specific to that job.

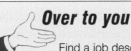

Over to you

Find a job description of potential interest to you. With a highlighter pen, mark the key skills that you feel the employer is looking for. Compare these skills with the five skills you have just listed and try to identify similarities.

Career history

Itemise each step of your career, starting with the most recent. Emphasise the aspects of your previous employment that most relate to the job you are applying for. If you are finding it difficult to make links between previous jobs and the one you are applying for, look at the job descriptions and see if there are any common themes. Nearly all types of employment need you to use communication skills or be able to work as part of a team, and these abilities are an integral part of health care.

To present your career history you need to have the following information:

● Dates should be listed with a 'from' and a 'to' e.g. '1999-present', '1997–1999' and should be either in the margin or ranged underneath each other so they are easy to read

● Brief address of employer (name and city is sufficient)

● Job title, including a brief description of your role and responsibilities (no more than four lines).

Achievements and results

This is a good section in which to sell yourself – it is the part that employers will be looking at with most interest. You may feel that you did not achieve a great deal in your last job but there is always something you have achieved. Be creative but stick within the realms of truth – remember you may have to answer questions on statements within your CV.

There are various ways in which this section can be divided – you can include your achievements within your career history, under each related job, or you can keep them as a separate section. There is no right or wrong, but if you worked somewhere and did not achieve a great deal compared to your other jobs, this is quite obvious when your achievements are integrated with your career history. If you have a separate section you do not need to state to which job your achievements relate. You can also subdivide your achievements in bullet-point headings. This is very effective if you have achieved in areas related to your new job description – clinical, management, professional, etc. Your employer can see at a glance what you have achieved in each subject-specific area.

It is also useful to remember the process of 'assess, plan, implement and evaluate' when listing achievements and results. This provides comprehensive proof of how you managed to achieve something. For example, 'Assessed need for change in off duty, discussed with colleagues and planned shift change, implemented new off-duty scheme and evaluated change through discussion with colleagues; new off-duty pattern adopted by manager'. Other useful verbs to use to describe your achievements are 'created' or 'designed'.

Education and qualifications

Education and qualifications can be separate headings depending on the breadth and depth of your education. As with career history, list your education starting with your most recent qualification and work backwards. Include:

- Dates – from and to
- Name of school, university or establishment
- Qualifications gained.

Professional development

Professional development can incorporate a description of how you have used your key skills to develop. You may wish to slightly expand upon how one of your achievements has complemented your professional development. Training courses or conferences are also included in this section, although training can be linked to education or qualifications, depending on the type of training. For example, training in basic life support from a recognised training provider would be better placed under qualifications, as the training has been substantial enough to give you a recognised skill. Do not list all the study days you have attended, just the ones relevant to the job you are applying for. Include:

- Dates – from and to
- Type of training/conference title
- Trainer provider/conference organiser.

Key points Top tips

When presenting your CV:

- Make sure you use a font that is easy to read such as Times New Roman or Arial and do not change font.
- Do not use a type size smaller than 11 points.
- Use bold to emphasise your name, attributes and skills.
- Ensure that your spelling is accurate (remember do not write 'I' or 'me').
- Your CV needs to be packed with verbs and adjectives.
- Make sure all the information is accurate and is presented logically.
- Use top-quality paper for printing – it makes all the difference.
- If you still do not feel confident producing your own CV you can access various websites or companies who will charge to produce one for you.
- Depending on how much space you have left on your CV you can state how the course/conference influenced your practice.

Top tips

- Do not include references unless asked to (this will give you more space).
- If you are including your CV with an application form there is no need to include your referees, as these will be listed on your application form.
- You can include interests and hobbies if you feel they are relevant. Often if you are applying for a course or first job, including interests and hobbies is useful as they give the employer an overview of your interests and potential capabilities, especially if you have little prior work experience.

Job application forms

A surprisingly large number of job applicants do not complete their application form correctly. The majority of application forms come with clear instructions and you need to follow the instructions exactly. If they ask for the application form to be handwritten, write it by hand; if they ask for experience or education to be listed in a certain way, list it in the way asked. These are basic instructions but can often be missed through oversight or rushing. An employer needs to know that you can follow basic instructions.

A job application form is similar to your CV in terms of presentation. Think of the job application form as an advertisement. This is your chance to market yourself to a potential employer – you want to make them want you. The whole process of getting a job is a marketing exercise, from the CV through the job application form to the interview itself. You need to present yourself in the best light at all times and you have to convince your new employer that you are the best person for the job. Don't be shy or modest – this is a time to show your skills and attributes.

Current role/post/job

When you are asked to describe your current role, look at your job description for headings, such as 'clinical' or 'management'.

Additional information

This is your best chance to sell yourself. This part of your application form provides the evidence for all the skills and attributes you claim to have. You do not need to provide evidence for every skill – select the more advanced skills and those you feel are most relevant to the job.

Sample CV

Sally Smith
1 Sally Smith Street, Sally Smithville, SS1 1SS
Telephone: 0111111111 E-mail: s.smith@*smithville.co.uk

An energetic, self-motivated individual with a keen interest in health care
A resourceful team worker with excellent interpersonal skills, now seeking a more challenging role within a dynamic Trust.

Personal details
Date of Birth: 13/01/76
Married
Full, clean driving licence

Career history
Current post:

Bebetter Trust, Smithville	2001 – present

Junior Sister F grade Surgical Services

- Providing evidence-based care to patients
- Supporting patients and their families
- Supporting G grade in their role
- Supervising staff and students
- Contributing to professional development of staff
- Link nurse to university students and postregistration course
- Responsible for off duty and management of subsequent issues
- Resource management
- Responsible for policies and protocol development

Staff Nurse E grade Surgical Services	1999–2001
Staff Nurse D grade Medical Services	1998–1999
Wards Trust, Jonesville	
Staff Nurse D grade Rotation Programme	1997–1998

Achievements

- **Successfully implemented primary care on an acute surgical ward with 25 patients. Evaluated introduction of primary care by administering questionnaires to all staff within the multidisciplinary team.**
- **Designed and produced an introductory booklet for new members of staff and students; this has been well received on the ward and a similar format is being produced by other wards within the Trust.**

Education and qualifications

University of Jonesville		1994–1997
BNurs (Hons) Nursing 2:1		
NMC	**PIN No.** 9711111S **Exp.** 05/06	
King Jones VI School, Jonesville		1987–1994
A Levels	Biology, General Studies	
GCSE	Mathematics, Biology, English Language, English Literature, French	

Professional development

'Equal Opportunities'	Bebetter Trust	2002
'Manual Handling Risk Assessment'	Bebetter Trust	2002
'Individual Performance Review'	Bebetter Trust	2001
'An Introduction to Primary Nursing'	Prime Trust 3-day conference	2000

Attending this conference enhanced knowledge and enabled networking with Trusts practising primary nursing, which facilitated the project undertaken.

'How to nurture a culture of change'	Altering Trust 1-day conference	2000

- Keep the section on your current role/post/job brief.
- Use bullet points as this makes the form easy to read.
- Choose aspects of your role that promote the skills you need for the new job.
- Look at the current role description on your CV and make sure your two descriptions match – you can copy it directly but you may have room to include more detail on the application form.
- Do not write 'see CV' in the 'current role' space; this can be extremely irritating for potential employers, who want all the information on the application form rather than having to flick between two sheets of paper.
- Try to avoid using an additional piece of paper – extra sheets can get lost and the application form looks neater without any extra pieces of paper.

Be succinct: look at the skills and attributes you have listed under 'current role' and try to provide examples of how they have developed or how you use them. For example, under 'current role' you may have put 'provides evidence-based care'. You can demonstrate this by writing under additional information

> On joining the oncology ward, experience from a different Trust had demonstrated that oral care in cancer patients improved when teeth were brushed twice daily and adequate hydration was ensured. On further reading and production of a paper critiquing current research, the ward altered its protocol on oral care; this change is currently being audited.

This extra information gives the employer an insight into your skills and how you have used them.

Ensure that what you have written is accurate and that you are happy to discuss each point, as your additional information will probably provide the basis of at least one of the questions at interview. Your portfolio should assist you in providing evidence for your skills and attributes. It will also satisfy any requests for evidence at interview.

Employers will sometimes ask for you to bring your portfolio to an interview, especially if you are newly qualified. There are many different health-care training providers and your portfolio will allow your potential employer to assess your training and what you have achieved.

Reflective activity

Look at the skills and attributes you have listed in your CV or that you think you possess. Consider how you would provide evidence of the skills and how you use them in your current practice.

Key points | **Top tips**

- Photocopy the application form so you can practise completing it and check how the completed form looks.
- If your writing is difficult to read, make sure you type your application form.

Covering letters

If you are submitting an application form, your covering letter need not be at all detailed. All the information about you will have been put in the application form. If you have typed your application form and your CV, your covering letter should be handwritten so that you can demonstrate your handwriting to the potential employer.

Key points | **Top tips**

- If your handwriting is difficult to read, try to write the covering letter as neatly as possible.
- Remember that, when accompanying an application form, the letter should be brief.
- Use high-quality, plain white stationery.
- Use the same paper to print your CV.

Sample covering letter

1 Sally Smith Street
Sally Smithville
SS1 1SS

Bebetter Trust
Smithville
SS1 2SS

Date

Dear _____

Re: Senior Sister Surgical Services, Ref: 5555

Please find enclosed my completed job application form and curriculum vitae. I look forward to hearing from you in the near future.

Yours sincerely,

S. Smith

Sally Smith

The interview and your portfolio

Always take your portfolio to interviews, even though you may not always have the time or opportunity to show it to the interviewer. If possible, carry extra copies of the assignments/reflections of which you are most proud (or those most relevant to that interview) so you can offer them to the interviewer to examine. This is vitally important if your portfolio is on CD-ROM, as not all interviewers will have the time or access to a computer during the interview to browse your portfolio.

You should use your portfolio to prepare for the interview, even if you do not get to share the contents of your portfolio at all during it. Reviewing the contents of your portfolio before an interview should provide you with fresh examples that you can draw from during the interview itself.

Key points | Top tips

- Please remember – your portfolio will not speak for itself or sell your skills to an interviewer; you have to do that. A good portfolio can be a big help, but in the end it must be you, not the portfolio, that proves your ability.

Over to you

You should now be aware of the best way to plan and present your CV. So, over to you! When you sit down to complete it, be organised – the following is a useful guide:

- Have the sample CV from this book by you.
- Find your current job description, to provide prompts for listing your current role responsibilities.
- If you are a student, obtain the aims and learning outcomes of the course you are studying (these are generally in your student handbook), as these will act as prompts to provide an overview of what you have achieved while on your course.
- Have the job description of the job you are applying for to hand.
- Look at the completed exercise sheet from the first exercise in this chapter, which will list your five key skills and personal statement.
- Look through the job description and, with a highlighter pen, mark the key skills that you feel the employer is looking for.
- Photocopy the application form so you can practise completing it. That way you can assess the size of handwriting required to fit all the details in.
- Ensure that you have some top-quality stationery at hand for your CV and covering letter.

Rapid recap

Check your progress so far by working through each of the following questions.
1. What is the purpose of a CV?
2. Make a list of the headings your CV should include.
If you have difficulty with either of the questions, read through the section again to refresh your understanding before moving on.

8

Portfolio examples

You should now feel happier as to what the portfolio should contain and look like, and which model to follow, whether reflective, incorporating Goodman's levels or within a continuing professional development model. You have been given various reflective and continuing professional development models from the literature to consider. You now need to decide which best suits you and how you are going to use it.

The three examples included in this chapter show how you can structure your portfolio and what evidence you can put in it. Each is examined from the point of view of both student and practitioner. They are cross-referenced to the chapters discussing the theories supporting the evidence for inclusion. None of the suggested lists of criteria is exhaustive and I would suggest that you consider some of the following points for each proposed section of your portfolio:

- What existing experience and knowledge do I already have that I can demonstrate in this section?

- What are the implications for me within this section, personally and professionally?

- What practical examples can I bring to this section to demonstrate my skills and competence?

- What sources of information can I draw upon to inform this section?

- What support from the literature can I provide for the evidence I have for this section?

- How can I demonstrate best practice in this section?

- What further development do I need to consider within this section?

Portfolio example 1

Preliminary pages

- **Contents/index page**
- **Introduction** – include a brief introduction to your portfolio, covering how you feel about it and whether you feel you've grown as a practitioner having compiled it
- **CV** (see Chapter 7)

Section 1: Professional and ethical practice – Contents

For student: You can further divide this section by splitting it into years. For each year of training you should include an entry from the suggested options.

For qualified practitioner: You can further divide this section into jobs. For example, if you are on a Trust staff nurse rotation you could include an entry from the following suggested criteria for each ward/unit, or you could divide the section into Benner's levels from novice to expert. As you begin the job, you are a novice and you can include an entry from each of the suggested criteria through each level to demonstrate development.

Suggested items to include

- Reflective entries relating to professional and ethical practice, using an identified reflective model and demonstrating reflective growth by using Goodman's levels of reflection (see Chapter 2)
- Assessment of practice documents relating to professional and ethical practice (student)
- Attendance at study days, workshops, lectures and seminars relating to professional and ethical practice, including information on how attendance has informed your practice
- Personal development plan and self-assessment that identifies learning needs for professional and ethical practice, and an action plan for how you propose to develop, including resources and time scale required (see Chapter 5)
- Essays, critical incidents or case studies relating to professional and ethical practice, with an explanation for their inclusion in this section (student)
- Consider the implications of professional and ethical practice for you personally and professionally
- Personal activities that relate to you and who you are and how you develop (see Chapter 2)

Section 2: Care delivery – Contents

For student: You can further divide this section by splitting it into years. For each year of training you should include an entry from the suggested options.

For qualified practitioner: You can further divide this section into jobs. For example, if you are on a Trust staff nurse rotation, you could include an entry from the suggested options for each ward/unit, or you could divide the section into Benner's levels from novice to expert. As you began the job, you were a novice, and you can include an entry from each of the suggested options for each level, to demonstrate development.

Suggested items to include

● Reflective entries relating to care delivery using an identified reflective model and demonstrating reflective growth by using Goodman's levels of reflection (see Chapter 2)

● Assessment of practice documents relating to care delivery (student)

● Attendance at study days, workshops, lectures and seminars relating to care delivery, including information on how attendance has informed your practice

● Personal development plan that identifies learning needs for care delivery, and an action plan for how you propose to develop, including resources and time scale required (see Chapter 5)

● Essays or written work relating to care delivery, with an explanation for their inclusion in this section (student)

● Personal activities that relate to you, who you are and how you develop (see Chapter 2)

Section 3: Care management – Contents

For student: You can further divide this section by splitting it into years. For each year of training you should include an entry from the suggested options.

For qualified practitioner: you can further divide this section into jobs e.g. if you are on a Trust staff nurse rotation you should include an entry from the following suggested criteria for each ward, or you could divide it into Benner's levels from novice to expert. As you began the job you were a novice and you can include an entry from each of the suggested criteria through each level to demonstrate development.

Suggested items to include

- Reflective entries relating to care management, using an identified reflective model and demonstrating reflective growth by using Goodman's levels of reflection (see Chapter 2)
- Assessment of practice documents relating to care management (student)
- Attendance at study days, workshops, lectures and seminars relating to care management, including information on how attendance has informed your practice
- Personal development plan that identifies learning needs for care management, and an action plan for how you propose to develop, including resources and time scale required (see Chapter 5)
- Essays or written work relating to care management, with an explanation for their inclusion in this section (student)
- Examples of care plans and an explanation of why you have included them in your portfolio
- Personal activities that relate to you, who you are and how you develop (see Chapter 2)

Section 4: Personal and professional development – Contents

For student: You can further divide this section by splitting it into years. For each year of training you should include an entry from the suggested options.

For qualified practitioner: You can further divide this section into jobs. For example, if you are on a Trust staff nurse rotation, you could include an entry from the suggested options for each ward, or you could divide the section into Benner's levels from novice to expert. As you began the job you were a novice, and you can include an entry from each of the suggested options through each level to demonstrate development.

Suggested items to include

- Reflective entries relating to personal and professional development, using an identified reflective model and demonstrating reflective growth by using Goodman's levels of reflection (see Chapter 2)
- Assessment of practice documents relating to personal and professional development (student)
- Attendance at study days, workshops, lectures and seminars relating to personal and professional development, including information on how attendance has informed your practice

- Personal development plan that identifies learning needs for personal and professional development, and an action plan for how you propose to develop, including resources and time scale required (see Chapter 5)
- Essays or written work relating to personal and professional development, with an explanation for their inclusion in this section (student)
- Personal activities that relate to you, who you are and how you develop (see Chapter 2)
- Learning style inventory and subsequent analysis (see Chapter 2)

The suggested options are by no means exhaustive; there are many other aspects of practice and representations of your development that you can include in the different sections. There are various lists throughout the book giving suggestions for material that can be readily incorporated into any of the above sections.

Portfolio example 2

Portfolio development and continuing professional development are obviously interlinked, as the portfolio is usually the medium in which you record your continuing professional development. This begins the moment you start your professional training. A brief look at Benner's model of skills acquisition might be useful as a model for your portfolio structure.

In her model, Benner (1984) identifies five levels, which adapt themselves very well to portfolio sections. You would therefore use the following structure.

Preliminary pages
- **Contents/index page**
- **Introduction** – include a brief introduction to your portfolio, covering how you feel about it and whether you feel you've grown as a practitioner having compiled it
- **CV** (see Chapter 7)

Section 1: Novice
Suggested items to include
- Reflective entries relating to the title of the section, e.g. reflecting on being a novice practitioner, using an identified reflective model (see Chapter 2)

- Assessment of practice documents relating to being a novice, e.g. year 1 (student)
- Attendance at study days, workshops, lectures and seminars relating to being a novice practitioner, including information on how attendance has informed your practice
- A personal development plan that identifies learning needs for the novice stage of practice, and an action plan for how you propose to develop, including resources and time scale required (see Chapter 5)
- Essays or written work relating to being a novice learner, e.g. year 1, with an explanation for their inclusion in this section (student)
- Work-based projects and research that reflect the novice level, e.g. the first time you were involved in a work-based project or research, when you were relatively inexperienced in the process
- Personal activities that relate to you, who you are and how you develop (see Chapter 2)

Section 2: Advanced beginner

Suggested items to include

- Reflective entries relating to the title of the section, e.g. reflecting on being an advanced beginner, using an identified reflective model (see Chapter 2)
- Assessment of practice documents relating to being an advanced beginner, e.g. year 2 (student)
- Attendance at study days, workshops, lectures and seminars relating to being an advanced beginner, including information on how attendance has informed your practice
- Personal development plan that identifies learning needs for this section and action plan on how you propose to develop, including resources and time scale required (see Chapter 5)
- Essays or written work relating to being an advanced beginner, e.g. year 2, with an explanation for their inclusion in this section (student)
- Work-based projects and research
- Personal activities that relate to you, who you are and how you develop (see Chapter 2)

Section 3: Competent

Suggested items to include

- Reflective entries relating to the title of the section, e.g. reflecting on being a competent practitioner, using an identified reflective model (see Chapter 2)
- Assessment of practice documents relating to being a competent practitioner, e.g. year 3 (student)
- Attendance at study days, workshops, lectures and seminars relating to being a competent practitioner, including information on how attendance has informed your practice
- Personal development plan that identifies learning needs for this section, and action plan on how you propose to develop, including resources and time scale required (see Chapter 5)
- Essays or written work relating to being a competent learner, e.g. year 3, with an explanation for their inclusion in this section (student)
- Work-based projects and research
- Personal activities that relate to you, who you are and how you develop (see Chapter 2)

Section 4: Proficient

Suggested criteria

- Reflective entries relating to the title of the section, e.g. reflecting on being a proficient practitioner, using an identified reflective model (see Chapter 2)
- Attendance at study days, workshops, lectures and seminars relating to being a proficient practitioner, including information on how attendance has informed your practice
- Personal development plan that identifies learning needs for this section, and action plan on how you propose to develop, including resources and time scale required (see Chapter 5)
- Evidence of contributing to or adhering to clinical governance, government legislation, professional body requirements, national and local policy
- Work-based projects and research
- Personal activities that relate to you, who you are and how you develop (see Chapter 2)

Section 5: Expert

Suggested items to include

- Reflective entries relating to the title of the section, e.g. reflecting on being an expert practitioner, using an identified reflective model (see Chapter 2)

- Attendance at study days, workshops, lectures, seminars or presenting at study days, workshops, lectures, seminars relating to being an expert practitioner including information on how attendance/presentation has informed your practice

- Personal development plan that identifies learning needs for this section, and action plan on how you propose to develop, including resources and time scale required (see Chapter 5)

- Evidence of contributing to or adhering to clinical governance, government legislation, professional body requirements, national and local policy

- Work based projects and research

- Personal activities that relate to you and who you are and how you develop (see Chapter 2)

- Publications and conference presentations

Benner's model is a good structure for a portfolio, as it continues through the transition from student to qualified practitioner. Remember, even when qualified, you will return to being a novice in some areas of your practice. This can seem a bit strange, as you may be experienced in reflection at Goodman's level 3 but the reflection may be on an area of practice that you are new to, which still means you are a novice practitioner. The levels are related to your experience as a practitioner not your experience at reflecting.

Within each section, you would be best to structure your material chronologically using periods of time appropriate to your development. The suggested options for inclusion are by no means exhaustive; there are many other aspects of practice and illustrations of your development that you can include in the sections. The portfolio inventory in Chapter 3 includes content suggestions that can be readily incorporated into any of the above sections.

Portfolio example 3

Preliminary pages

- **Contents/index page**
- **Introduction** – include a brief introduction to your portfolio, covering how you feel about it and whether you feel you've grown as a practitioner having compiled it
- **CV** (see Chapter 7)

Section 1: Development and change

Suggested items to include

- Reflective entries relating to section title, e.g. reflecting on being an expert practitioner, using an identified reflective model (see Chapter 2)
- Attendance at study days, workshops, lectures and seminars, or presenting at a study day, workshop, lecture or seminar
- Provide evidence that promotes best practice
- Provide evidence of ensuring that policies and practices for care are based on evidence
- Personal development plan that identifies learning needs for development and change, and action plan on how you propose to develop, including resources and time scale required (see Chapter 5)
- Evidence of consideration given to auditing the care received by clients
- Evidence of integration of good practice into the work environment and of supporting colleagues to do the same
- Evidence of contributing to or adhering to clinical governance, government legislation, professional body requirements, national and local policy

Section 2: Developing appropriate clinical skills

Suggested items to include

- Reflective entries relating to the development of appropriate clinical skills, using an identified reflective model and demonstrating reflective growth by using Goodman's levels of reflection (see Chapter 2)
- Provide evidence of development of a personal culture that promotes 'learning from experience' to ensure improvements in practice (see Chapter 2)

- Provide evidence of progress towards acquisition of the necessary skills listed in job description (see Chapter 6)
- Provide documented evidence of a framework for measuring achievement and evaluating effective performance
- Evidence of contributing to or adhering to clinical governance, government legislation, professional body requirements, national and local policy
- Attendance at study days, workshops, lectures and seminars or presenting at a study day, workshop, lecture or seminar, with specific relevance to enhancing of skills

Section 3: Education and learning

- Reflective entries relating to education and learning, using an identified reflective model and demonstrating reflective growth by using Goodman's levels of reflection (see Chapter 2)
- Provide evidence of development of a personal culture that promotes 'learning from experience' to ensure improvements in practice
- Attendance at study days, workshops, lectures and seminars relating to education and learning, including how attendance has informed your practice
- Personal development plan that identifies learning needs for education and learning, and an action plan on how you propose to develop, including resources and time scale required (see Chapter 5)
- Essays or written work relating to education and learning, with an explanation for their inclusion in this section (student)
- Personal activities that relate to you, who you are and how you develop (see Chapter 2)
- Learning style inventory and subsequent analysis (see Chapter 2)

Section 4: Research and dissemination

- Provide evidence of work-based projects that enhanced client care
- Provide evidence of client care being guided by evidence-based practice
- Evidence of contributing to or adhering to clinical governance, government legislation, professional body requirements, national and local policy
- Provide evidence of research and its dissemination

As with the Benner model, each section would be best structured chronologically using periods of time appropriate to your development. The possible options suggested within each section are by no means exhaustive – there are many other aspects of practice and evidence of your development that you could include. The portfolio inventory in Chapter 3 includes content suggestions that can be readily incorporated into any of the above sections.

Reference

Benner, P. (1984) *From Novice to Expert: Excellence and power in clinical nursing practice*. Addison-Wesley, Menlo Park, CA.

Appendix

Rapid Recap – answers

Chapter 1

1. What is a portfolio?

A collection of individual material to provide proof of personal growth, continuing professional development, life-long learning and competence.

2. What is a profile?

A public version of the portfolio – a summary of your portfolio that can be offered at interview to support your application or submitted to professional bodies as proof of continuing professional development.

3. What is the purpose of keeping a portfolio for:

a)   a health-care student

b)   a qualified practitioner?

a)   A portfolio is often used in professional development and is assessed as part of a health-care student's education and training.

b)   The UKCC brought in legislation in 1995 that individuals on the professional register must maintain a personal professional profile. The profile is proof to the NMC that you, as an individual practitioner, are keeping yourself updated, maintaining competence and remaining accountable for your actions.

Chapter 2

1. What are the four dimensions in Kolb's Learning Cycle?

Concrete experience (getting involved)

Reflective observation (listening)

Abstract conceptualisation (creating an idea)

Active experimentation (making decisions).

2. What is 'deep learning'?

When you integrate all the information you have received, through teaching sessions, observing practice, participating in practice, reading and discussions, and develop a deeper understanding of the key issues. You can then use this knowledge at a later date and apply it to different situations, thus enabling problem-solving.

3. According to Schon, what is the difference between reflection-in-action and reflection-on-action?

Reflection-in-action is a dynamic process, the intuitive art of 'thinking on your feet', which occurs while practising and influences the decisions made and care given. Reflection-on-action is a retrospective process, which occurs after the event and contributes to the development of practical skills.

Chapter 3

1. What key questions should you consider each time you want to put a piece of evidence into your portfolio?

a)   What existing experience and knowledge do I already have that I can demonstrate for this piece of evidence?

b)   What are the implications for me, personally and professionally?

c)   What practical examples to demonstrate my skills and competence can I bring to this piece of evidence?

d)   What sources of information can I draw upon to inform this piece of evidence?

e)   What support can I find in the literature for this piece of evidence?

f) How can I demonstrate best practice in this piece of evidence?

g) What further development do I need to consider for this piece of evidence?

2. **List five things you have to remember in order to produce a well-organised paper portfolio.**

a) Buy a good quality cover

b) Use acetate or plastic sleeves to display and protect materials

c) Use clear referencing if one piece of evidence informs one or more sections in your portfolio

d) Include a table of contents

e) Label and index material.

Chapter 4

1. **Explain the difference between a formative and summative assessment.**

To assess something formatively usually means that the results do not count towards deciding that a student has failed or passed a module or programme of study. For instance, formative assessments may be undertaken early in a module to provide students with essential diagnostic feedback about their performance and what needs to be done to correct weaknesses and build upon strengths. Summative assessments determine whether students are awarded their degree or diploma, or whether they fail.

2. **List four sets of modifying factors that assessors should take into consideration when assessing a student's portfolio.**

Any of the following:

- Specific module/programme/course-related criteria against which the portfolio was developed and against which it should be assessed

- The portfolio developer's own individualistic portfolio development criteria, balanced against module/programme/course-determined portfolio development requirements, including specific learning outcomes

- Special considerations listed by the portfolio developer to be taken into account

- A note of special self-acknowledged limitations experienced in the process of the portfolio development and/or in the final portfolio product

- A list of the portfolio developer's personal and professional development and learning needs

- Any specific skills, competencies, forms of knowledge and attitudes the student set out to achieve within the context of self-development through portfolio building.

3. **What are the notions of accreditation of prior learning (APL) and accreditation of prior experiential learning (APEL)?**

Under APL, health-care professionals may be able to seek and gain recognition for previous learning. Under APEL, they may also be able to seek accreditation for prior experiential learning (learning on the job through experience).

Chapter 5

1. **How is the specific purpose of practice development defined at Addenbrooke's NHS Trust?**

To ensure that all care is:

- Centred on the client (not the needs of the staff)

- Based on evidence (i.e. based on published data, good practice guidelines and feedback from patients)

- Appropriate for the needs of each patient

- Effective.

2. **Name the three categories of life-long learning.**

Theoretical, personal and practice.

3. **What is clinical supervision?**

A practice-focused professional relationship that enables you to reflect on your practice with the support of a skilled supervisor. Through reflection you can further develop your skills, knowledge and enhance your understanding of your own practice.

4. **Why do health-care professionals need to incorporate professional development into their role?**

In order to remain competent, relevant and clinically effective.

Chapter 6

1. **What do the following represent?**
   a) **Learning for practice**
   b) **Learning while practising**
   c) **Learning through practice**

   a) Theory and education, which includes professional development courses/modules and study/theory days.

   b) Experience, which includes personal and professional development through reflection, personal development plans, reflection in action and reflection on action.

   c) Evidence-based practice and literature, which includes evidence-based practice and practice-based projects/research.

2. **When you qualify, what should you do with your student portfolio?**

   Do not start a brand new portfolio when you qualify, you need to elicit the key factors about yourself from your student portfolio to inform your personal development plans and subsequent professional career.

Chapter 7

1. **What is the purpose of a CV?**

   The main purposes of a CV are to:
   - Attract an employer's interest by being well designed and attractive to look at
   - Provide interesting and relevant information
   - Sell your key strengths and attributes.

2. **Make a list of the headings your CV should include.**

   There are no set rules on what a CV should include, but suggested headings are:
   - Personal details
   - Attributes and skills
   - Career history (most recent first and work backwards)
   - Achievements while in post or in previous posts
   - Education and qualifications
   - Professional development.

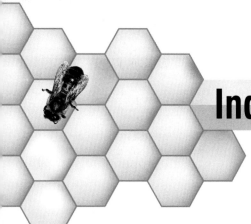

Index